The Phoenix's Guide To Self Renewal

A Daily Food Diary and Exercise Journal

To guide, motivate and inspire you on your weight loss journey.

Melissa Alvarez

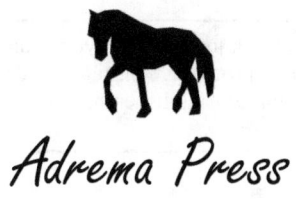

A NOTICE TO THE READER
The ideas and suggestions contained in this book reflects the opinion of the author based on her own experiences and are not intended as a substitute for psychological counseling or consultation with your physician. This book is not a medical guide or a diet program. It contains motivational chapters and journal for logging progress. All matters regarding your health require medical supervision. The author and publisher assume no liability for damage resulting from this books information. Consult your doctor before beginning any weight loss or exercise program to determine the best program and activity level for you.

Copyright © 2001 by Melissa Alvarez
All Rights Reserved.
www.MelissaA.com *or* www.MelissaAlvarez.com

Second Edition
ISBN: 1-59611-036-8
ISBN 13: 978-1-59611-036-6

All Rights Reserved. Except for use in any review, the reproduction or utilization of this work in whole or in part in any form by any electronic, mechanical or other means, now known or hereafter invented, including xerography, photocopying and recording, or in any information or retrieval system, is forbidden without the prior written permission of both the publisher and copyright owner of this book.

First published 2001 by New Age Dimensions

Cover Design by Melissa Alvarez
Published by arrangement with the author.

First Trade Paperback Printing: June 2004
10 9 8 7 6 5 4 3

> If you purchased this book without a cover, you should be aware that this book is stolen property. It was reposted as "unsold and destroyed" to the publisher, and neither the author nor the publisher has received any payment for this "stripped book."

Are you a Phoenix?
Do you wish to renew yourself?
Do you have determination, desire, and courage?
Then you too can succeed!

This book is for anyone with a true desire to change his or her current situation. If you have suffered with your weight and are determined to reshape your body then this is the book for you. It is a straightforward, strong approach to body transformation while empowering you on an emotional and spiritual level. This book is not a weight loss program but a motivational guide to keep you on track as you progress with your chosen weight loss plan.

Dedicated to:

You and Me!
Because we deserve it!

Acknowledgments

For those who wrote to me asking if I had any of my personal copies of this book left in stock – thank you. Your numerous emails and letters are the *only* reason I've released this title again.

I'm smiling at all of you!

Regarding This Second Edition

When *The Phoenix's Guide To Self Renewal* was first published in 2001, it was 416 pages (six months of journaling) and I literally printed the books in my home, burning out numerous printers and copiers due to the demand. If you have one of those first editions it's a collector's item. A three month comb bound version was printed in 2004 when I expanded New Age Dimensions into a small press. In 2006 it was taken out of print when New Age Dimensions closed its doors. In the past few months, I have had numerous requests for this title so I've revised the book and am releasing the second edition.

The reviews for *The Phoenix's Guide To Self Renewal* were very positive, however, there were a few complaints as well. While it's impossible to please everyone, the formatting comments were taken into consideration in this new edition. I also want to reiterate that this book is a journal with ten motivational chapters. This **IS NOT** a weight loss program. While I've shared my experiences, I recommend that you contact your physician prior to beginning any weight loss program and then use this book to keep track of your progress or to motivate you when you're feeling down. I hope you enjoy this new edition of *The Phoenix's Guide To Self Renewal*. I wish you the best on your weight loss journey.

Sincerely,

Melissa Alvarez

Contents

Chapter 1: Why I wrote this book   9

Chapter 2: The Myth of The Phoenix   15

Chapter 3: Set your Goals   18

Chapter 4: Motivation   22

Chapter 5: Renewing Your Spirit   26

Chapter 6: Choosing a weight loss program   29

Chapter 7: Your Personal Trainer   32

Chapter 8: Strategies for Success   35

Chapter 9: Lifetime Maintenance   39

Chapter 10: Daily Journal   41

Chapter 1
Why I wrote this book

Hello! Welcome to an open minded and blunt approach to weight loss and the renewal of your frame of mind about your body. This book is not loaded with technical jibber jabber you can't understand because I don't talk or write that way. It's a no-nonsense, motivational approach to weight loss from someone who went through it and is going through it again. I'm not inventing some new diet scheme but trying to provide insights and techniques that are useful and beneficial to you, and me, as we go down this path together. The chapters in this book ARE NOT a diet program; rather, they are a motivational philosophy written to inspire you on your weight loss path. I wrote this book for me but I decided to share it with you. Let's have fun along the way!

So why did I write this book? After the birth of my first son, I had suffered with weight problems. Before I got pregnant with him, at my heaviest I was only 125 lbs., which wasn't bad because I'm 5'8" tall. I was supposed to be at my goal by my birthday but guess what folks? I didn't make it. I was honestly sick and tired of looking the way I did and sincerely wanted to do something to change my appearance. Three weeks before my birthday, I started looking for a journal to purchase and use as I progressed along my path of weight loss.

My search was in vain. I wanted a journal where I could log food intake and exercise together. All the journals I found were either a food journal or exercise journal. None of them offered a place for me to vent if I had a bad day or pat myself on the back if I had a great day. If they did, all the spaces where you were supposed to write were tiny. Who writes that small anyway? Certainly not me, I wanted space, I wanted it easy and I wanted it now. And there were none to be found. So I decided to make my own journal. I've always read that the people who have the most success with losing weight and keeping it off write down what they do on a daily basis. I absolutely hate writing down every piece of food I put in my mouth all day and counting calories and all that kind of stuff so I wanted something extremely easy and efficient.

By using my own motivation, my own journal, my own tactics and sticking with it, I lost a total of thirty-five pounds and kept it off for three years. Unfortunately, we went through a bad period of time and the weight crept back on. So here I am again – right here with you, doing what I did when I first released this book back in 2001 – tracking my weight loss and I strive to get back down to my goal weight. I did it before and I can do it again – so come on – let's do this together!

Back then, I also realized that if I had looked for a journal that would meet all my needs and was unable to find one maybe others were having the same problem. So I decided to publish this book. I didn't expect to sell as many as I did. My first print run was sold out in two weeks. And during the first two and a half months that the book was on the market it sold almost a thousand copies, was in the top three hundred in sales on Amazon.com where it also received rave reviews. Since its original release back in 2001 it has sold nearly four thousand copies. Not bad for a self-published book. I sincerely hope you find it as useful as I did.

You're probably wondering why all of this is in a chapter instead of an introduction. Well, if you're like me, and you may or may not be, you'll skip over the intro and jump right into chapter one. I wanted you to read this because I feel it is important. I also want you to know at this point I gained back some of the weight I lost and I'm still striving toward my goal of 130 but I've never given up. And no, I'm not a wonder case who has lost 5000 lbs in a day. Just kidding, but you know what I mean. I have a family to take care of and life gets in the way with me just as it does with most people. When I get sidetracked or disgusted with my progress, I read these chapters again - for motivation. So, you can use whatever diet plan works best for you; use this journal to keep track of your progress and the chapters for motivation when you need them.

When I started out I was 95 pounds overweight at a whopping 225 at 5'8" tall. I had a Body Mass Index of 34 and have brought it down to a 29. My body fat percentage was 50% and is now 35%. I don't have as much to lose this time but I'm leaving these stats here from the first edition. Why? You're probably wondering what woman in her right mind would put all her statistics out here for the whole world to see, especially when they are so bad. I mean, let's face it people – half of my body was FAT!!! Call me crazy but you know what I just did? I admitted it to myself by writing it down. I faced the fact I let myself go for too long and haven't succeeded in getting back to my pre-pregnancy weight because I kept looking in the mirror and saying, "I don't look that bad – I'm tall, I can hide it". Well, guess what? I couldn't hide it. I was just fooling myself into believing I could hide under baggy clothes. Now I'm not fooling myself any longer. I've admitted my size to myself and to the world and it is the first major step we all must take in order to succeed - seeing ourselves as we really are and not as we imagine ourselves to be.

I believe you too can obtain your goals if you have the desire, determination, and motivation to face yourself.

I have come to the realization that weight loss does not have to be an all or nothing kind of thing. I mean, how many of us have starved ourselves for weeks just to have a bad day and say the heck with all of this! I've been good for weeks so I deserve a little treat! And then we do it – we eat everything in sight and feel like crap afterwards. I'm sure there is some medical term for this but I call it giving up. That's right – we give up and when we give up we eat and eat and eat and eat and eat. And why do we do this?

Because we lose control, feel like a failure – like we just

didn't have the will power to do what we know deep in our hearts we should do – stop after just a taste. Because that dang sugar called our names – loudly and with passion! That bread just smelled so darn good we just couldn't help ourselves, and besides it was just a "little" treat. That is, until it got out of hand, and then we find ourselves rolling in self-pity and depression because of what we just did to our body and our weight loss efforts.

Ok, so we just made ourselves sick. Too much food at one time will do that to a person you know. Really, too much of anything will do that to a person. Think about it – too much alcohol – sick. Too many spins on a ride at the fair – sick, too much salsa dip – sick, too many chocolate covered strawberries – well, maybe I'm getting carried away here but you get the picture. We should do everything in moderation. When we don't, we feel bad in some way. Whether it's a physical sickness like a hangover or an emotional thing like being depressed because we just inhaled a box of cookies when we were going to eat just one.

There is something you can do. You can change the way you think about the actions you take in your life and discover your reasons for taking these actions. By looking deep inside yourself you can find the answers you seek.

Diet – let's take a look at that word. What is meant by diet anyway? We all know it is what a person or animal eats. Break it down – diet: die-t, di-et, d-ie-t. The dictionary says diet is a controlled intake of food and drink designed for weight loss, for health or religious reasons, or to control or improve a medical condition. Diet is used to describe a food or drink that is intended for people trying to lose weight, usually because it is low in calories or fat, or contains a sugar substitute. Well to me diet means that you will die trying (die-t), or Di was an ET (di-et), or Did I eat that? (d-ie-t). I think we should take the word diet out of the language. Instead of diet let's call what a person does when they try to lose weight a Teid (Tee-id), the exact opposite of diet, which stands for "to eat is divine" or "to exercise is delightful." Let's eat interesting, healthy foods on a daily basis, add in some exercise that will benefit our bodies and return to our true shape and weight. That sounds like a recipe for success, doesn't it?

We don't have to die trying or feel like we're going to die while we are improving our lifestyles. Diets are usually setups for failure. You really have to change your thought processes and lifestyle in order to be successful in losing weight and keeping it off.

Yeah, yeah, yeah, I know you're heard that crap before but you know what? It's true. If we are going to lose this weight and keep it off we have to change the way we think about things, the way we approach food, and the way all of our thoughts and feelings affect our self-image. It's the only way to make it work. There is no quick fix, no easy way out, no magic pill – no matter how bad we want those things to be true. It's just us - our mind, our determination, our willpower and our ability to look at ourselves, really look at ourselves and see what it is we want to change in our lives. Then we just have to do whatever it takes to achieve that goal. We have to realize this is something we have to do for ourselves. You have to put yourself first - before the kids, husband or wife, job, and all the other things that are involved in your daily life. Take time for yourself, decide if you need to do this and if your answer is yes, then just do it. Don't make excuses because then you're only cheating yourself.

You are not going to be able to do this by sheer willpower alone, if you try, you will be constantly thinking about food and feeling like you are giving up something you deserve. Instead, build a support team around you. Tell your family and friends you are going on a Teid. Ask them to refrain from offering you foods that you've decided not to eat even if it's a "special occasion". Tell them you need their support, love and encouragement. When you say "no thanks", you mean it, and pressure isn't appreciated. Another good idea is to join a support group. Whether it's a weight-loss center that offers weekly counseling, an online site, a group who gathers to talk about weight loss, or just a friend you can call whenever you feel like you're going to stray from your plan; any time you can share your efforts with others, the easier it will be to accomplish your goal.

The hardest part of our success is getting started and having a positive support team. You know as well as I do, people who are not trying to change their lives or their weight will unconsciously sabotage our best efforts. Yeah, we may have to address this issue more than once in our lives but so what? This is my second time around but hey- life happens – it's not all or nothing. The great thing about it is that we can lose the weight again – and again, and again, and again if we have too. That said, yo-yo dieting isn't a good idea so try to keep the weight off once you lose it. A friend of mine says she "drops" the way because if you "lose the weight" it might find you again. That's a great mindset!

Spouses may not always understand and although they may think they are being helpful it may not seem that way to us. If you have Internet access, there are a lot of websites that offer free or paid services which include chat rooms and support groups where you can go to mingle with others who are on the same path. You can discuss topics and feelings you may not feel comfortable discussing with those closest to you, but can discuss with someone who is in your same shoes.

Weight loss is a tough road to walk. There will be times when you'll gain back pounds that were previously lost. Hey, that's just a fact of life even though we might not like it. I'm at that point right now. What they say about weight lost being harder as you get older is definitely true. It sucks but that's the way it is. During times when you get off track or have a situation that puts your diet on the back burner, or any number of things that can mess up your new eating plan, try to use motivation as a key to regaining your focus on your goals and getting back on track. Then you too will succeed.

Chapter 2
The Myth of The Phoenix

The myth of the Phoenix Bird is associated with the sun god in ancient Greek and Egyptian mythology and is symbolic of immortality, resurrection and life after death.

According to mythology only one Phoenix Bird could exist in our world at a time. It was a fabulous bird and was said to be as large as an eagle, with brilliant crimson and gold feathers and a harmonious song. It lived for a very long time; ancient writers gave it a life span of at least five hundred years and up to one thousand four hundred sixty one years.

The Phoenix lived in Paradise, a land of indescribable beauty lying beyond the distant horizon towards the rising sun. Death doesn't exist in Paradise and after 500 or more years passed, the Phoenix became weary and wished to die. In order to achieve this goal the Phoenix had to fly into the mortal world and to the scented spice groves of Arabia where it collected aromatic herbs and continued its flight to the coast of Phoenicia in Syria. Upon arrival it found the highest branches of a palm tree and built a nest out of the collected herbs and aromatic wood then looked towards the east to wait for the new dawn, which would bring death to the Phoenix.

As the sun rose, the Phoenix faced its death with a beautiful song that caused the sun god himself to stop and listen to the bird's melody. Some say that as he moved his chariot forward a spark from the hooves of his horses would set the Phoenix's nest on fire; others say that the bird would set the nest on fire by itself. Either way the Phoenix was consumed by the flames and died.

A new Phoenix miraculously emerged from the ashes of the dead Phoenix. It embalmed the ashes of the deceased Phoenix in an egg of myrrh and flew with it to Heliopolis, the city of the sun, and placed the egg on the altar of the sun god.

That's such a great story. It has always inspired me. I believe we all have the ability to reinvent ourselves just as the Phoenix has the ability to renew itself from its ashes.

Let's just pause for a moment and reflect on this mysterious bird. How are we like the Phoenix? The Phoenix lives in a land of beauty. Well, I think we live in a land of beauty – it may not always be paradise but it is beautiful. Death is definitely a reality here. I believe we need to think of death not in terms of a physical death as the Phoenix experiences, but as a symbolic death.

If we let our old ways of eating die within ourselves and we celebrate the death of the old ways of thinking and the birth of the new stronger thoughts and desires within us, then we have a new agenda for life, and we shall succeed. We have let the fire of our eating burn out of control for too long. Let's harness the power of the flames, control it and turn it into our passion. Take the energy of the fire and focus it on changing our attitudes about weight loss and actually losing the weight. Can you feel the power of your passion? I know I'm on fire and I feel we too can rise again from the flames of disappointment, despair and failure to soar in the renewed spirit within ourselves. We too can miraculously emerge from the ashes of our old selves to realize a new transformed self. The Phoenix is a symbol of rebirth and life after death. I say we think of it as a rebirth in our thinking and the life of a new transformed body as we say goodbye to the body we have been unhappy with for so long.

So what else makes us like the Phoenix? The Phoenix had the desire to die. It wanted death because it was weary and tired from living for such a long time. I don't say that we want death – no one wants to physically die but aren't we tired just like the Phoenix? Tired of carrying around excess weight?

Tired of not being able to do the kinds of things that we really yearn to do? Tired of wishing we were skinnier? Tired of saying "When I lose weight I'm gonna do so and so." Tired of being unhappy with our selves and letting that unhappiness affect all other areas of our lives? I know I am. Are you tired too? Do you have the desire? Are you ready to do this for yourself and no one else? I decided to do this for myself. I hope you join me on this path.

    You too can be like the Phoenix and experience a new life after allowing the obstacles of the current life to die and be reborn as new thoughts, a new strength of conviction and a faith in yourself and your success.

Chapter 3
Set your Goals

So what are your goals? What do you hope to achieve out of your chosen weight loss program? I know you're probably saying, "Duh! WEIGHT LOSS dingbat!!!!!" But what else will you achieve? Maybe it's a healthy, toned, drop dead gorgeous body; maybe it's a new car (yeah you read that right! I say if you lose a lot of weight you deserve something new that's just for you! Selfish? Maybe. Motivation? Most definitely!) Maybe it's the success that you will feel once you have accomplished your goals.

Whatever your desires you can achieve them, but you have to set your goals down in black and white before you start so that you will have something to work toward. This is a given in the business world. No bank will give a loan to a business without a business plan. The most successful people write down goals that they wish to accomplish and work toward those goals. Without goals we would be doing what… wandering aimlessly along through life just existing on a daily basis and probably bored to tears. Goals make things fun. Without goals we wouldn't go anywhere in life. Who hasn't planned a vacation, a night out on the town or a nice romantic dinner? Those are all goals. Things we plan and then strive to accomplish in order to fulfill our desires.

How do we go about setting a goal and accomplishing it? I believe that there are several things we need to do in order to be successful and I call it POWVIP. So what does that stand for you ask? *Passion, Overcome, Write, Visualize, Imagine* and *Persist*.

In order to achieve your goals you have to be passionate about reaching those goals. There has to be a strong desire from within you to achieve the goals you set. If you don't desire it with a *Passion*, then you will not achieve it because your heart will not be in what you are doing. You'll just be so-so about the project, which in this case will be weight loss, and not passionate about it. It is the passion that fuels us, that pushes us forward that makes us consider all options before we progress. For instance, if you are passionate about losing weight then before you pop that chip into your mouth you will think, "Is this going to help me attain my goal or hinder me from achieving it?" When you consciously think about what you are doing because you're passionate about it, then you will more than likely put the chip back in the bag?

It's at times like these when you will *overcome* your obstacles. How do you recognize your obstacles? Do you eat when you are mad? How about for comfort? Are you using the food to hide your true feelings regarding the situations in your life? Is it easier to eat then to face the real problem? These are examples of some of the obstacles you might encounter on your journey. Once you realize your passion, and then think about what obstacles you may encounter while you are trying to attain this goal. An obstacle can also be a learning tool. For example, if you know you eat when you are mad or depressed, try to take a walk when you feel that way instead of heading for the kitchen. You'll find the fresh air and movement will not only clear your head but also channel your emotions to something other than eating. By meeting the obstacles head on you will be able to confront and overcome them.

Write all of this down. Write down your passions, your obstacles, what goals you are trying to attain and how you envision yourself attaining them. Make a game plan. You don't see football players entering the field without a game plan or a businessman entering a meeting without an agenda, and you shouldn't set off on this adventure without a strategy. So put it down on paper. Make a list of why you want this – the more reasons you have the more passionate you will be about attaining your goal. List your obstacles and how you plan on overcoming them. Use this as a reference tool for yourself if, a month down the line, you forget why you are doing this or have lost any of the enthusiasm that you had at the beginning of this quest. Review your goals whenever you need inspiration. Give yourself a time frame to complete your goal. Try a long-term goal of one year and make your short-term goals for each month within that year. If you need to lose 70 lbs in the year to reach your goal then you should lose about 6 pounds each month. As long as you lose those 6 pounds, you have reached the goal for that month and have scored a major accomplishment! If you lose more- great! If it's less, then just try harder next month.

Visualize and *imagine* what you will achieve. Visualize your body as healthy and vibrant. Imagine yourself without all the excess weight. Visualize how you will feel. How do you present yourself to the world? Are you more confident? Are you happy? How do you look? Are you healthy? Toned?

Take time each day of this journey to sit quietly for a few minutes and visualize what you are working toward and imagine yourself reaching your goal. What do you want to achieve from these goals you have set forth for yourself? Now see yourself achieving these goals and how you look and feel once you have reached your goal. Has your life changed? Is it better? Worse? The same? Look toward the future and realize what you are working for by embarking on your journey. You are a very important person. Look within yourself; see just how important you are, and give yourself the credit that is yours.

Be *Persistent*. It is persistence that will get you to the goal you have set. It is very easy to give up on your goals. You can get sidetracked at any time but it will be your persistence that will bring you back to center and get you back on track. Persistence is something the successful use to get ahead. If the president of a company just said, "Oh the heck with this, I'm tired of trying" then he wouldn't be the president of that company would he? You have to think the same way. I can do this, I will do this, I deserve this and I'm going to get what I desire. Be persistent and you will reach your goal and realize you are a POWVIP:

POWERFUL, VERY IMPORTANT PERSON!

Chapter 4
Motivation

What motivates you? What will keep you on track? What makes you do the things that you do? When you figure that out you can also figure out what is keeping you from losing the weight you want to lose.

Let me just tell you a little about my motivation for trying to finally succeed with my weight loss efforts. Maybe some of what I'm saying will seem familiar to you. Maybe it will seem totally alien to you. But either way, hopefully, you will see what motivation is and how we can apply it on a daily basis. Let's start with a little of my background.

I am a work at home Mom with three children. I've owned my own business for the last 10 years. I have been overweight since 1992 when I gave birth to my first son. I was 30 years old and weighed between 115 and 130 pounds my entire life when suddenly I gained 10 pounds for apparently no reason. I didn't know at that time I was pregnant so I tried to lose it. No matter what I did I just kept gaining. Due to my body producing low levels of the pregnancy hormone at the beginning of my pregnancy, it took six weeks to find out that I was expecting. By that time I had gained almost 25 pounds. Well, now I was eating for two and boy did I eat for two. That is such a bunch of malarkey anyway. You're not really eating for two; you just need to eat healthy for the sake of your unborn baby. I took it to mean that it was a free for all and I could eat anything in as large or as small of a quantity that I wanted for the next 7 months. By the time the baby was born I had gained 67 pounds and went into labor at 197 pounds. Afterwards, I dropped weight very easily and was soon down to 160 – not at goal but significantly smaller than when I gave birth. But it didn't last. By the time I got pregnant with my second baby I had gained up to 180. I only gained 30 pounds with this pregnancy but that put me up at 210. By the time he was weaned I had only dropped back to 197. Two weeks after that I discovered I was pregnant again. With my third child I gained 22 lbs and was back at 197 right after the birth. But for some reason, I felt like I was gaining after I had him but I didn't dare step on a scale.

When I finally did I was shocked to see I weighed 225 pounds. I weaned him soon after and started trying to lose. I'd lose some and gain it back, lose it and gain it back again. It was a vicious cycle. So what motivated me to lose weight?

The biggest motivating factor for me was my fortieth birthday. I couldn't believe that I was already at this age and had children between the ages of 9 and 1. Amazing. When I looked in the mirror I no longer knew myself. My face was round, not the square angular face that I used to have. My body looked like it was falling apart and no matter how beautiful my husband said I was; I just felt like a humongous whale. Then I noticed my 3 year old was starting to gain weight and he only wanted to drink milk and eat sweets. He was starting to trade regular food for only sugary foods. That made me realize he was picking up my bad habits. I know kids who are overweight have a hard time in life and I didn't want that to happen to my child. To top it all off, I was looking at things in my attic and found a box of clothes that said "Melissa size 9/10", so I decided to look inside. What a reality check that was for me. Some of my favorite outfits were in that box, outfits I used to wear when I first started dating my husband. I held them up to me and was absolutely shocked to see I was twice the size I used to be. The waist on some of these dresses was the size of my thigh now. I held the side of the dresses up to my side, stretched it over me, and the other side of the waist hit my belly button. I was utterly disgusted. I couldn't believe what I was looking at in the mirror. I hadn't, up until that moment, realized how large I had actually gotten. These clothes were a kick in the butt for me. I needed to do something and I needed to do it now. If I had increased that much in size there was no telling what was going on inside my body. I have low blood pressure naturally but what else was going on in there? To add more power to the punch of this reality check, in walks my 9 year old while I'm holding up one of the dresses and asks me whose clothes did I have? When I told him that they were my old clothes his eyes got as big as saucers and he said, "Oh my gosh Mom! You've gotten FAT!!"

So I decided to take drastic actions. I was now completely and totally motivated to do something about my weight. Geez, how many times did I have to be shown what was happening in my life before I did something about it? I no longer even owned a bathing suit. I was uncomfortable dancing in front of anyone and hid my true, adventuresome, happy self behind a quiet, unhappy, overweight person. It was time to change.

So that was my motivation to lose weight when I first published this book. In the time since, I've gained back some weight and my motivations are similar but not the same. You see, this time around I'm not losing weight for the vanity part of it – for wanting to look the way I did before having children. That's a fantastic motivator but this time I'm doing it for my health. Time passes quickly whether we like it or not. I'm not getting any younger. Now is the time to rid myself of the unhealthy habits I've picked up over the years and to get my weight back where it was after the original release of The Phoenix's Guide. I hope to have quite a few years left here on this planet and it's never too late to live a healthy life.

Take some time to look inside yourself, to be completely honest with yourself, to think of the reasons you want to lose weight and write it all down. There's space right here in this book just for your motivations, obstacles and goals. Just remember, this path will be something you choose to do, something you truly want just for you. Not to impress someone else, not because you're told you need to do it, not because your spouse wants you to be skinnier, but because you are unhappy with the way you look and you want to lose weight for yourself. Because you want more energy, want to be healthier, and want to feel great! Because you are the most important person in the world and you want to take care of this one body that you have so you don't have knee pains, hand pains, back pains and all the other pains associated with being overweight. Do this because you want to do it just for yourself, your health, and your self-esteem.

Chapter 5
Renewing Your Spirit

What is the spirit? Let's go again to the dictionary and see what it says. Spirit is defined as a supernatural being that does not have a physical body, for example, a Ghost, Fairy, Angel. Nope - that's not the one I was looking for hang on a second. Ok, found it! Spirit is the vital force that characterizes a living being as being alive; it is a person's will, sense of self, or enthusiasm and energy for living, somebody's attitude or state of mind. Well, that says a lot doesn't it?

So why would we want to renew our spirit? In my case it was because I had a very negative conception of my body, I had been skinny my whole life until I had children. Now I wouldn't exchange having children for being skinny for anything in the world, but having those little angels wreaked havoc on my body, especially the last two which came back to back. When I tried to lose weight I did it without trying to change the way I thought about my body first. I'd diet, lose a little, and keep at that vicious cycle but never really lose more than 5 or 10 pounds because deep in my heart I felt I really didn't deserve to be skinny again. Why did I feel this way? Who the heck knows? I sure didn't, I just knew it was hard to lose weight and after every little accomplishment I sabotaged myself and went right back to my old ways of eating. My spirit wasn't happy. I hadn't accepted myself as the person I had become, and because of that, I couldn't start down the path of true transformation.

I believe that until we accept ourselves as we are right now, this very minute, with every little bit of cellulite, every piece of flab, every bump, line and wrinkle, then we will not be able to move forward. Self-acceptance is the first step in transforming ourselves. We have to see where we are now and where we have been in order to see where it is we are going. That is what is different with me this time. This time I looked at myself in a different way. I accepted the fact I had gained all this weight and it was time to start following my heart and not my head. In my heart I truly wanted to be back at my ideal weight and it was my stupid head that kept telling me I could never do it and I'd always look this way. This time I told my head to shut up and listened to my heart for a change.

I could have cried as I looked at my reflection in the mirror that day and accepted myself. I had gained so much weight, I now looked like two of the person that I once was. My body was flabby, not firm, and I had become my worst nightmare. As I stood there looking at myself in my big, baggy clothes, I accepted what I had done to myself and decided I had walked as far down this road as I wanted to go. It was time to turn around and go home. It was time to become myself again. To stop eating like a maniac, to accept that I had done this to myself because I kept shoving the food in my mouth and sitting my butt on the couch and not moving or working out. Now, that's a hard thing to do you know. It's so easy to blame everything and everyone else in the world, except yourself, for being overweight. Yes, some people do have health problems and should lose weight under a doctor's care but a lot of us just eat too darn much. That was my problem and once I realized that I couldn't blame anyone else except myself, something just seemed to click within me. I had accepted the fact that in the past I didn't have the passion to do something about my weight and decided to change right then.

When we look deep within ourselves and take note of the things that are the hardest part of ourselves to look at, then we are truly renewing our spirit. We are giving ourselves back the vital force, the enthusiasm; the will and the sense of self we need to carry forth on a new adventure to achieve a new goal.

If we don't let go of the negative energies before we start this process, then once you meet your weight loss goal you'll be skinny and unhappy. You'll still feel those negative feelings about yourself even though you may have lost a great deal of weight. So wouldn't it be better to face yourself and let go of these negativities now before you start? I know it was a difficult thing for me to do and it will be hard for you too. But I'll tell you; I feel so much better about myself now that I have faced the truth and carried on. What is it they say? The truth shall set you free. Believe me it does. There's no way I would want to be my skinny self and still have all the negative thoughts I had about myself. I would still be miserable and that's not the point of all of this. The point is to be healthy, happy and a positive person. So think about it and decide if you too would be happier by changing the way you think about yourself before you begin.

Also, accept the fact that you will have times where Mr. Negativity will pop in your brain and start nagging away at you. At times like these just tell that stupid thought you're no longer thinking about this with your mind, but are feeling this with your heart. You don't need those negative opinions of yourself resurfacing, you choose to ignore them and realize what a great thing you are doing for yourself. Remember too that when you think of things in a negative manner, you're drawing negativity to you. Don't do this. Think positive thoughts, imagine yourself at your end goal and strive toward that goal. Negativity will only hold you back whether it's coming from those around you or from within yourself. Positivity rocks! Use it.

Once we have renewed our spirits we are free to embark on any journey we desire.

Chapter 6
Choosing a weight loss program

So now you've written down your goals, you have your motivation, you're passionate about losing weight, and you've faced yourself and renewed your spirit. Now what? This is the point where you will choose which kind of weight loss program is right for you.

There are lots of weight loss programs out there. High protein, low protein, high carbohydrate, low carbohydrate, rice diets, grapefruit diets, diets for sugar addictions and carbohydrate addictions, herbal diets, diet pills, soup diets, miracle diets, percentage diets, fad diets and just about any other kind of diet that you can imagine with new ones coming out all the time. Which kind of diet is right for you? That's a hard thing to say and is something you will have to determine for yourself. I can tell you what regime I follow and if it makes sense to you then feel free to try it too. You have to choose a diet plan that will allow you to eat a variety of foods and is healthy. Not every plan will work for everyone so as you review the various plans out there keep a couple of things in mind. Is the plan simple and easy to follow? Does it sound appealing to you? Is this plan something you feel you can stick with or do you feel you'd get tired of eating like this after several weeks? Remember, this is a journal with motivational chapters – not a weight loss plan – you'll have to find that at a bookstore or weight loss center near you!

I recommend that you stay away from fad diets, single food diets, pills, and anything that seems unhealthy to you. I have tried every single diet under the sun but never had any success because as soon as I went back to my "normal" way of eating I gained the weight back. Little did I realize then, my "normal" way of eating sucked and I was eating in the unhealthiest way of all. Once I renewed my spirit, I realized this was the case and came up with a plan of my own invention that is working well for me. I'll explain it in this chapter. I also recommend that before you start any weight loss and/or exercise program that you consult with your physician.

Reading various types of diet programs and trying all kinds of plans enabled me to see the kind of things that seemed healthy, things that appealed to me, and things I didn't like. I have learned I am hopelessly addicted to refined sugar and giving it up was going to be one of my hardest obstacles. Coffee loaded with sugar in the mornings had been a staple of my diet for years and that was going to have to change. I did research and found I needed to have some starch, veggies, protein, fruit, dairy and a little fat each day to eat a well balanced diet. I could eat between a 1200 and 1500 calorie a day diet without having to measure every item and still lose weight. I decided to stay within this range so my body didn't go into starvation mode from having too few calories. I also read in several different places that calories eaten in the morning are rarely converted to fat. Sounded like a good idea to me, so I decided to make breakfast my biggest meal of the day, eating as much as I wanted while staying within my serving allotments for the day. Lunch and dinner would be smaller and lighter than breakfast and use whatever daily allotments were left. Sometimes I will even drink a premixed diet shake for dinner. To know exactly how many servings I was eating, I looked on the container or I counted one half of a cup of veggies, one piece of meat the size of the back of my hand when I made a fist, or one pat of butter as a serving. I used one of my kid's plates that had three sections in it for food and the alphabet around the edge. It was smaller so it looked like I was eating a full plate of food when in fact I was eating much less. And I practiced my ABC's at the same time! I also decided my last meal would be between 6:00 and 7:00 o'clock at night and I would drink tons of water and green tea all during the day. Both help keep you feeling full and green tea is a natural diuretic and metabolism booster. Sodas both diet and regular were going to be history (another hard obstacle for me) and I was going to exercise before breakfast every morning. I'd read that exercising before breakfast caused your body to burn more stored fat as fuel since you hadn't eaten since the previous night. Plus, I take a multivitamin daily.

And that's what worked for me. It's very simple, easy to do and healthy and I'm seeing results for the first time ever.

Chapter 7
Your Personal Trainer:
Get your butt off the couch and move!!!!

Don't you just hate this part??? Exercise. It's the elixir of health but who the heck wants to sweat and hurt, gasp for air and be sore the next day just to get healthy? No pain no gain they say. Well whoever said that was out of their mind in my opinion. I could walk from here to the ends of the earth, but to do an aerobic type of exercise. Forget it!

It's amazing what forcing yourself to do something will do to your state of mind. The first week you're cussing out the guy or girl on the video while you're trying to figure how just how the heck they move like that. You're yelling out in pain because you can't breathe and shooting darts from your eyes at your kids as they fall on the floor laughing at you. Then by the second week you're keeping up a little better and breathing easier and now the kids think it's fun to jump around with Mommy. By week three it's become a habit. You have to get those forty-five minutes of aerobics in each morning because it makes you feel so much better and it gives you a great start to your day. By now the kids could care less and you're just trying to not jump on them as they run around under your feet.

So what kind of exercise is best? I believe that doing a variety of exercises helps to keep you interested in the entire concept of exercise. If you only do the same thing over and over, day after day, week after week, pretty soon you're going to hate it and you'll just stop. That's not what you want to accomplish with exercise. The point is to get your body-moving if only a little bit. I have always been able to walk two to six miles pushing one hundred pounds of kids and a double stroller and not even be sore the next day. But to do an aerobic exercise just killed me. I could barely lift my legs, my stomach would cramp up after a few sit-ups and I was just dying. But believe me it does get better as your body gets used to being tortured. I'm just kidding about the tortured part but you will become adjusted to the workouts and actually start to enjoy them. This is where *persistence* comes into play.

I started out with a variety of workout tapes I had accumulated over the years and had never used. I mixed and matched them so I would get a different type of workout each day. I chose tapes that were about forty-five minutes long and did them before breakfast. I really like the cardio kick boxing types of video's and the dancing ones. Step type of video's really turned me off because I have bad knees. I eventually narrowed my choices down to about four different tapes that I use on a rotating basis.

Now if you can join a gym, and know you will use the membership, then go for it. There are great classes offered in aerobics, jazzercise, spinning, yoga, boot camps and other areas as well as having the ability to do strength training at the gym. But you have to be able to afford the price of the membership and have the time to commit to going there on a daily basis. For me it was better to exercise at home because I have two small children. The one time I did join a gym it didn't work out for me because my kids would start crying in the middle of class every time and I didn't use the membership.

Each morning I do an exercise video or dance around my living room for forty-five minutes, or jump rope, or jump on my mini-trampoline. In the afternoons I try to walk. If I'm too tired I skip the afternoon walk because I know I have gotten in at least one forty-five -minute session that morning. I try to walk every day.

When I go out to the stores I park farther away so I have to walk a longer distance to get where I want to go. I take the steps instead of the elevator whenever possible. All of those kinds of things add up you know. And then I add strength training.

Now, if you have kids this will make sense to you but if you don't – sorry, you'll have to borrow somebody else's kids to do these exercises or buy some dumbbells to do them. When this book was first released, I'd take my eighteen-month-old (forty pounds) hold him across my arms and do curls. I hold my arms behind my head to do triceps exercises, put my hands together and my three-year-old (fifty lbs) grabs on and I lift him. Then I do crunches the regular way. For my legs I do kick backs, leg lifts and bicycle my legs in the air. I also put my knees to my chest and take turns lifting my kids with my feet on their stomachs. They pretend they are flying and my legs get an awesome workout. For my waist I take my broom, put it across my shoulders, sit on my coffee table and twist the waist from one side to the other, keeping my hips stationary. Those are some of my inventive ideas! Have fun coming up with some of your own.

Pick the type of exercises you like and do them. It can be anything you think you'll like to do as long as your body is in motion. You have to realize that in order to be successful with losing this weight and keeping it off you will have to move your body. There's no getting around it. It's a fact we just have to accept. If you think back to any point in your life when you weighed less, weren't you more active? When I was at my skinniest I would go out and dance for hours at a time, every single weekend. I loved dancing and it kept me in shape. That's why one of my choices for exercising is dancing around my house. It makes you feel great, lifts your spirits and is a great workout! So whatever your choices, stick with them, be persistent, and soon they will become a habit that you really enjoy.

Chapter 8
Strategies for Success

This chapter has concepts and ideas that have helped me as I try to bring out the Phoenix inside me and transform myself to my true shape. I hope they help you as well.

Always live like tomorrow will never come.

Don't put off until tomorrow what you can do today.

Give 100% of yourself in everything that you do - not only when you do something for others but when doing something for yourself too.

Try something new every week.

Close up the kitchen early.

Try to get at least eight hours of sleep each night.

Don't give up on yourself if you fall off your Teid (remember that's diet backwards) one day. Just jump right back in the next day. Don't let one small step backwards be the end of all the progress you've made so far. Write how you feel about the day on the journal page and then forget it. Start tomorrow as if yesterday never happened in regards to your slip from your program.

Drink lots and lots of water. Try using a thirty-two oz refillable bottle and drink two of those a day instead of eight glasses with eight ounces of water. It's easier to empty two larger bottles then eight smaller ones even though it's the same amount of fluid.

Drink green tea whenever you get hungry. It will make you feel full, is a natural diuretic and boosts your metabolism.

Skip on caffeine and artificial sweeteners.

When you feel hungry and it's not time for a meal, take a walk. It gets your body moving and will get rid of your hunger.

Are you often in a rush? Keep a supply of pre-mixed meal replacement shakes in the fridge so you can drink one of those instead of skipping your meal and bingeing later.

Never skip a meal, especially breakfast.

Keep a food and exercise journal.

Ignore others if they seem to be sabotaging your efforts. Don't let them get to you.

Do some kind of exercise daily.

Do this for YOURSELF!!

Smile! It uses more muscles than frowning; it's contagious and makes you feel great.

Hum a song.

Pick some flowers (or buy some).

Take a hot tub bath full of bubbles. Put some candles around the tub and just relax. While you're there meditate about your progress and congratulate yourself on what you've accomplished. Make mental notes on areas you want to try to improve upon.

Use your time walking to become more spiritual, meditate, or just contemplate anything that you want. There's nothing like the fresh air and nature to make you feel at one with the Universe.

Enjoy your life.

Tell the people that are important to you how much you love them every day.

Have fun in everything that you do.

Sweat!!!

Limit your fat intake.

Don't deprive yourself of any food. If you must have it, eat half the portion you would normally eat, enjoy it and forget about it. Remember to do everything in moderation.

Help a friend.

If you're bored find something to do other than to eat. Visit a website or send me a letter, write to a friend, walk, just do something that will get your mind off of food and eating.

Emotional eaters (I'm one!) – when your emotions get the best of you – do something physical, sweat it out but whatever you do, GET OUT OF THE KITCHEN!!!

Don't starve yourself by eating really small portions. Make sure that you eat the right amount of foods so that your body will not go into starvation mode.

Don't get impatient with yourself. It took a while to put the weight on and it's going to take a while to get it off too.

Release your negative body image and any negative thoughts that may keep you from being successful. Renew your spirit.

Enlist the help of a friend or join a support group. Make an agreement with someone who is willing to support you and call them whenever you feel like you are going to slip from the program. A positive voice encouraging you helps tremendously. Willpower alone is too difficult and you may not succeed. Get supporters in place first!

Be like the Phoenix. Transform yourself from the ashes of your old ways of thinking and your current weight to a new way of thinking and your true body image.

Chapter 9
Lifetime Maintenance

Look in that mirror. Like what you see? Umm hummm – what a fine, toned, hot body!

You did it!!!!! Let me be the first to congratulate you!!!

CONGRATULATIONS!!!!!!

I am so proud of you and the accomplishments you have made. You have set a goal for yourself and have achieved your goal. You are the Phoenix. You have transformed and renewed your mind, body and spirit. It is a great task you have completed.

So how do you maintain this new body you have worked so hard to achieve? You don't give up. You keep doing the same as you have always done. You might increase your food intake a little but make sure you monitor your weight for the next several months to make sure the foods you add are not causing you to put any of the weight back on. As you gradually increase your food intake you will find a comfortable medium where you know you can eat without gaining.

If you do see that you put on a few pounds at any time just go back to limiting your portions and increasing your exercise until you lose the weight. I feel that five pounds is the most you should let your weight increase once you attain your goal before you do something about it. I've seen so many people that I know lose lots of weight, work out and achieve an awesome body and within months of doing all of that they put it all right back on again and then some. Will you tell me what the point of that is? If you work your butt off to get the type of body you want, then why in the world would you not take the small amount of effort required to maintain it? You've already done the hardest part. It can happen though when you're not expecting it. Maybe you're going through a hard time financially or emotionally and the weight just creeps back on without you even realizing it. Well, then just know it's time to work your butt off again – literally – and get back on track to "drop" that weight that found you again. Thanks again to my friend for that saying! The same thing happened to me though it took almost five years to find me.

Another suggestion I have for maintaining your weight is to keep this journal, the one you've been writing in while you were on your weight loss path, as a reference book. When you put on a few pounds go back and read what you wrote when you had a LOT of weight to lose. How were you feeling then? Do you really want to go back to where you used to be? Do you want to feel that way again? If you do then go right ahead and eat as much as you want until you gain the weight back, but if you don't like what you see in yourself on those pages, then put down the fork and pick up an exercise video or go for a walk.

No one ever said this would be an easy path to follow. Nor will it ever get any easier even when you are at your goal. The older you get the harder it is to lose weight. That sugar will always call my name but now I can ignore it if I so choose.

You have succeeded and have risen to the challenge put before you.

I commend you.

Chapter 10
Daily Journal

    I wrote this book and designed the diary and journal to fit my needs and to motivate me as I lost weight. This daily journal has worked quite well for me. I hope it works well for you. Start each day with the date and your weight. If you choose to only weigh weekly just put an X there until you get to your weigh-in day.

    All you need to do is check off your servings as you eat them. Remember these are the servings that you will eat for the entire day so spread it out between meals. I also included a section for those of you who like to write down what you're eating during the day as well as a section for grams of fat, carbohydrates, fiber and calories for those of you who like to track that information. I hardly ever fill this in but sometimes it helps to look at what I've eaten over the course of a week and then make changes based upon any goof ups or things I notice that I should be doing differently.

    Next is the exercise section. Write down any exercise that you do. Whether it's a video, walking, or dancing around your house for an hour - put it down. It counts! If you do some type of aerobic activity plus weight training write it down. If you're not using weights but say you walked for a half hour and then did 20 leg lifts and 30 sit ups put the walking under aerobic exercise and the leg lifts and sit-ups under strength training or other exercise. Then on the opposite page is a section where you can write how you're feeling for the day. Did you stick to your goals? Did you totally screw up today? Are you irritated or hungry today? With this layout your whole day is right there in front of you, what you did on one side and how you felt about it on the other. Write it all down, praise yourself or vent your frustrations, release it on these pages so you can start all over tomorrow. Remember it's the long-term goal we're reaching towards.

Good luck on your journey! I wish you much success and would love to hear your thoughts on this journal and whether or not you found it useful. You can email me at contact@MelissaA.com.

MONTHLY PROGRESS CHART

Fill in this chart on the same day each month. If you start your weight loss program on the 12th then each month on the 12th you will complete the chart. Put your weight and the inches that each part measures and watch the numbers drop!

	Weight	Chest	Waist	Hips	Thigh	Calf	Forearm	Upper Arm	BMI
Month 1									
Month 2									
Month 3									
Month 4									
Month 5									
Month 6									
Month 7									
Month 8									
Month 9									
Month 10									
Month 11									
Month 12									
GOAL									

BMI

BMI stands for Body Mass Index. BMI is a measurement used by physicians who study obesity. It is a person's weight in kilograms divided by height in meters squared. Use the chart on the next page to calculate your BMI and enter it in the above chart.

BMI CHART

Underweight 18.5 or less
Ideal 19 – 24
Overweight 25-29
Obese over 30

BMI	19	20	21	22	23	24	25	26	27	28	29	30	35	40
Height							Weight							
4' 10"	91	96	100	105	110	115	119	124	129	134	138	143	167	191
4'11"	94	99	104	109	114	119	124	128	133	138	143	148	173	198
5' 0"	97	102	107	112	118	123	128	133	138	143	148	153	179	204
5' 1"	100	106	111	116	122	127	132	137	143	148	153	158	185	211
5' 2"	104	109	115	120	126	131	136	142	147	153	158	164	191	218
5' 3"	107	113	118	124	130	135	141	146	152	158	163	169	197	225
5' 4"	110	116	122	128	134	140	145	151	157	163	169	174	204	232
5' 5"	114	120	126	132	138	144	150	156	162	168	174	180	210	240
5' 6"	118	124	130	136	142	148	155	161	167	173	179	186	216	247
5' 7"	121	127	134	140	146	153	159	166	172	178	185	191	223	255
5' 8"	125	131	138	144	151	158	164	171	177	184	190	197	230	262
5' 9"	128	135	142	149	155	162	169	176	182	189	196	203	236	270
5' 10"	132	139	146	153	160	167	174	181	188	195	202	207	243	278
5' 11"	136	143	150	157	165	172	179	186	193	200	208	215	250	286
6' 0"	140	147	154	162	169	177	184	191	199	206	213	221	258	294
6' 1"	144	151	159	166	174	182	189	197	204	212	219	227	265	302
6' 2"	148	155	163	171	179	186	194	202	210	218	225	233	272	311
6' 3"	152	160	168	176	184	192	200	208	216	224	232	240	279	319
6' 4"	156	164	172	180	189	197	205	213	221	230	238	246	287	328

My Goals Are: _____

My Motivations: _____

My Obstacles: _____

Notes to myself:

Notes to myself:

Dance like no one is watching. ~ *Unknown Author*

Today was: _____

Success is the proper utilization of failure ~Unknown Author

Daily Journal   Today's Date: _____   Weight: _____
My Mood: _____

Extra checklist boxes are to accommodate for various weight loss programs. You can check the boxes, list individual foods under Today Was page, keep a numerical log below or do all three.

Checklist: Bread/Starch: ☐☐☐☐☐☐☐☐, Protein: ☐☐☐☐☐☐☐☐
Veggies: ☐☐☐☐☐☐☐☐, Fruit: ☐☐☐☐☐☐☐☐, Fat: ☐☐☐☐☐☐,
Dairy: ☐☐☐☐☐☐☐, Water (8oz): ☐☐☐☐☐☐☐☐☐☐, Vitamin ☐

What I Ate: Protein | Fat | Carbs | Fiber | Calories | Points | Other

	Protein	Fat	Carbs	Fiber	Calories	Points	Other
Breakfast:							
Lunch:							
Dinner:							
Snack:							
Other Meal							
Other Meal							
Add it up:							

Circle One
Daily

☺

😐

☹

Hunger Level

+   -

Exercise: (Include Videos, Walking, Exercise equipment, Any type of exercise that you did)
After exercising I felt _____
Type_____ How Long: _____
Type_____ How Long: _____
Type_____ How Long: _____
Type_____ How Long: _____

Strength Training: After working out I felt:_____

_____ X_____	Reps at _____	lbs
_____ X_____	Reps at _____	lbs
_____ X_____	Reps at _____	lbs
_____ X_____	Reps at _____	lbs
_____ X_____	Reps at _____	lbs
_____ X_____	Reps at _____	lbs
_____ X_____	Reps at _____	lbs
_____ X_____	Reps at _____	lbs

Keep your head and your heart going in the right direction and you will not have to worry about your feet ~ Unknown Author

Today was:

Happiness is a choice that requires effort at times ~ Unknown Author

Daily Journal   Today's Date: _____   Weight: _____
My Mood: _____

Extra checklist boxes are to accommodate for various weight loss programs. You can check the boxes, list individual foods under Today Was page, keep a numerical log below or do all three.

Checklist: Bread/Starch: ☐ ☐ ☐ ☐ ☐ ☐ ☐ ☐, Protein: ☐ ☐ ☐ ☐ ☐ ☐ ☐ ☐
Veggies: ☐ ☐ ☐ ☐ ☐ ☐ ☐ ☐, Fruit: ☐ ☐ ☐ ☐ ☐ ☐ ☐ ☐, Fat: ☐ ☐ ☐ ☐ ☐ ☐,
Dairy: ☐ ☐ ☐ ☐ ☐ ☐ ☐ ☐, Water (8oz): ☐ ☐ ☐ ☐ ☐ ☐ ☐ ☐ ☐ ☐, Vitamin ☐

What I Ate: Protein | Fat | Carbs| Fiber |Calories| Points | Other

Breakfast: ____|____|____|____|____|____|____   Circle One Daily

Lunch: ____|____|____|____|____|____|____   ☺

Dinner: ____|____|____|____|____|____|____   😐

Snack: ____|____|____|____|____|____|____   ☹

Other Meal ____|____|____|____|____|____|____   Hunger Level

Other Meal ____|____|____|____|____|____|____   +   -

Add it up: ____|____|____|____|____|____|____

Exercise: (Include Videos, Walking, Exercise equipment, Any type of exercise that you did)
After exercising I felt _____
Type_____ How Long: _____
Type_____ How Long: _____
Type_____ How Long: _____
Type_____ How Long: _____

Strength Training: After working out I felt:_____

_____	X_____	Reps at _____	lbs
_____	X_____	Reps at _____	lbs
_____	X_____	Reps at _____	lbs
_____	X_____	Reps at _____	lbs
_____	X_____	Reps at _____	lbs
_____	X_____	Reps at _____	lbs
_____	X_____	Reps at _____	lbs
_____	X_____	Reps at _____	lbs

When you reach for the stars, you may not get one, but you won't come up with a handful of mud, either ~ Unknown Author

Today was: _____

Failure is only the opportunity to begin again, this time more wisely ~*Unknown Author*

Daily Journal   Today's Date: _____   Weight: _____
My Mood: _____

Extra checklist boxes are to accommodate for various weight loss programs. You can check the boxes, list individual foods under Today Was page, keep a numerical log below or do all three.

Checklist: Bread/Starch: ☐☐☐☐☐☐☐☐, Protein: ☐☐☐☐☐☐☐☐
Veggies: ☐☐☐☐☐☐☐☐, Fruit: ☐☐☐☐☐☐☐☐, Fat: ☐☐☐☐☐☐,
Dairy: ☐☐☐☐☐☐☐, Water (8oz): ☐☐☐☐☐☐☐☐☐☐, Vitamin ☐

What I Ate: Protein | Fat | Carbs | Fiber | Calories | Points | Other

Breakfast: ____|____|____|____|_____|____|____   Circle One
                                                          Daily
Lunch: ____|____|____|____|_____|____|____
                                                           ☺
Dinner: ____|____|____|____|_____|____|____
                                                           😐
Snack: ____|____|____|____|_____|____|____
                                                           ☹
Other Meal ____|____|____|____|_____|____|____
                                                        Hunger Level
Other Meal ____|____|____|____|_____|____|____
                                                          +   -
Add it up: ____|____|____|____|_____|____|____

Exercise: (Include Videos, Walking, Exercise equipment, Any type of exercise that you did)
After exercising I felt _____
Type_____ How Long: _____
Type_____ How Long: _____
Type_____ How Long: _____
Type_____ How Long: _____

Strength Training: After working out I felt:_____

_____	X_____	Reps at	_____ lbs
_____	X_____	Reps at	_____ lbs
_____	X_____	Reps at	_____ lbs
_____	X_____	Reps at	_____ lbs
_____	X_____	Reps at	_____ lbs
_____	X_____	Reps at	_____ lbs
_____	X_____	Reps at	_____ lbs
_____	X_____	Reps at	_____ lbs

Whatever you do, do well, and may success attend your efforts ~ Unknown Author

Today was: _____

Excuses are the tools with which persons with no purpose in view build for themselves, great monuments of nothing ~ Unknown Author

Daily Journal   Today's Date: _____ Weight: _____
My Mood: _____

Extra checklist boxes are to accommodate for various weight loss programs. You can check the boxes, list individual foods under Today Was page, keep a numerical log below or do all three.

Checklist: Bread/Starch: ☐☐☐☐☐☐☐☐, Protein: ☐☐☐☐☐☐☐☐
Veggies: ☐☐☐☐☐☐☐☐, Fruit: ☐☐☐☐☐☐☐☐, Fat: ☐☐☐☐☐☐,
Dairy: ☐☐☐☐☐☐☐☐, Water (8oz): ☐☐☐☐☐☐☐☐☐☐, Vitamin ☐

What I Ate: Protein | Fat | Carbs| Fiber |Calories| Points | Other

Breakfast: _____|_____|_____|_____|_____|_____|_____   Circle One
                                                                Daily
Lunch: _____|_____|_____|_____|_____|_____|_____
                                                                 ☺
Dinner: _____|_____|_____|_____|_____|_____|_____
                                                                 ☹
Snack: _____|_____|_____|_____|_____|_____|_____
                                                                 ☹
Other Meal _____|_____|_____|_____|_____|_____|_____
                                                              Hunger Level
Other Meal _____|_____|_____|_____|_____|_____|_____
                                                                + -
Add it up: _____|_____|_____|_____|_____|_____|_____

Exercise: (Include Videos, Walking, Exercise equipment, Any type of exercise that you did)
After exercising I felt _____
Type_____ How Long: _____
Type_____ How Long: _____
Type_____ How Long: _____
Type_____ How Long: _____

Strength Training: After working out I felt:_____

_____	X _____	Reps at _____	lbs
_____	X _____	Reps at _____	lbs
_____	X _____	Reps at _____	lbs
_____	X _____	Reps at _____	lbs
_____	X _____	Reps at _____	lbs
_____	X _____	Reps at _____	lbs
_____	X _____	Reps at _____	lbs
_____	X _____	Reps at _____	lbs

Forget mistakes. Organize victory out of mistakes ~ Unknown Author

Today was: _____

Give yourself a compliment today and really listen ~ Unknown Author

Daily Journal   Today's Date: _____   Weight: _____
My Mood: _____

Extra checklist boxes are to accommodate for various weight loss programs. You can check the boxes, list individual foods under Today Was page, keep a numerical log below or do all three.

Checklist: Bread/Starch: ☐☐☐☐☐☐☐☐, Protein: ☐☐☐☐☐☐☐☐
Veggies: ☐☐☐☐☐☐☐☐, Fruit: ☐☐☐☐☐☐☐☐, Fat: ☐☐☐☐☐☐,
Dairy: ☐☐☐☐☐☐☐, Water (8oz): ☐☐☐☐☐☐☐☐☐☐, Vitamin ☐

What I Ate: Protein | Fat | Carbs| Fiber |Calories| Points | Other

Breakfast: ____|____|____|____|____|____|____

Lunch: ____|____|____|____|____|____|____

Dinner: ____|____|____|____|____|____|____

Snack: ____|____|____|____|____|____|____

Other Meal ____|____|____|____|____|____|____

Other Meal ____|____|____|____|____|____|____

Add it up: ____|____|____|____|____|____|____

Circle One
Daily

☺

☺

☹

Hunger Level

+   −

Exercise: (Include Videos, Walking, Exercise equipment, Any type of exercise that you did)
After exercising I felt _____
Type_____ How Long: _____
Type_____ How Long: _____
Type_____ How Long: _____
Type_____ How Long: _____

Strength Training: After working out I felt:_____

_____ X _____	Reps at _____	lbs
_____ X _____	Reps at _____	lbs
_____ X _____	Reps at _____	lbs
_____ X _____	Reps at _____	lbs
_____ X _____	Reps at _____	lbs
_____ X _____	Reps at _____	lbs
_____ X _____	Reps at _____	lbs
_____ X _____	Reps at _____	lbs

Everywhere you go there are angels in disguise ~ Unknown Author

Today was: _____

Take time for yourself every day ~ Melissa Alvarez

Daily Journal Today's Date: _____ Weight: _____
My Mood: _____

Extra checklist boxes are to accommodate for various weight loss programs. You can check the boxes, list individual foods under Today Was page, keep a numerical log below or do all three.

Checklist: Bread/Starch: ☐☐☐☐☐☐☐☐, Protein: ☐☐☐☐☐☐☐☐
Veggies: ☐☐☐☐☐☐☐☐, Fruit: ☐☐☐☐☐☐☐☐, Fat: ☐☐☐☐☐☐,
Dairy: ☐☐☐☐☐☐☐, Water (8oz): ☐☐☐☐☐☐☐☐☐☐, Vitamin ☐

What I Ate: Protein | Fat | Carbs| Fiber |Calories| Points | Other

Breakfast: ____|____|____|____|____|____|____   Circle One Daily

Lunch: ____|____|____|____|____|____|____   ☺

Dinner: ____|____|____|____|____|____|____   😐

Snack: ____|____|____|____|____|____|____   ☹

Other Meal ____|____|____|____|____|____|____
                                                        Hunger Level
Other Meal ____|____|____|____|____|____|____
                                                           +   -
Add it up: ____|____|____|____|____|____|____

Exercise: (Include Videos, Walking, Exercise equipment, Any type of exercise that you did)
After exercising I felt _____
Type_____ How Long: _____
Type_____ How Long: _____
Type_____ How Long: _____
Type_____ How Long: _____

Strength Training: After working out I felt:_____

_____ X_____ Reps at _____ lbs
_____ X_____ Reps at _____ lbs
_____ X_____ Reps at _____ lbs
_____ X_____ Reps at _____ lbs
_____ X_____ Reps at _____ lbs
_____ X_____ Reps at _____ lbs
_____ X_____ Reps at _____ lbs
_____ X_____ Reps at _____ lbs

Today is brighter because I care ~ Melissa Alvarez

Today was: _____

For problems, sweat is a good solvent ~ Unknown Author

Daily Journal   Today's Date: _____   Weight: _____
My Mood: _____

Extra checklist boxes are to accommodate for various weight loss programs. You can check the boxes, list individual foods under Today Was page, keep a numerical log below or do all three.

Checklist: Bread/Starch: ☐☐☐☐☐☐☐☐, Protein: ☐☐☐☐☐☐☐☐
Veggies: ☐☐☐☐☐☐☐☐, Fruit: ☐☐☐☐☐☐☐☐, Fat: ☐☐☐☐☐☐,
Dairy: ☐☐☐☐☐☐☐, Water (8oz): ☐☐☐☐☐☐☐☐☐☐, Vitamin ☐

What I Ate: Protein | Fat | Carbs | Fiber | Calories | Points | Other

Breakfast: ____|____|____|____|____|____|____   Circle One
                                                        Daily
Lunch: ____|____|____|____|____|____|____
                                                          ☺
Dinner: ____|____|____|____|____|____|____
                                                          😐
Snack: ____|____|____|____|____|____|____
                                                          ☹
Other Meal ____|____|____|____|____|____|____
                                                     Hunger Level
Other Meal ____|____|____|____|____|____|____
                                                        +   -
Add it up: ____|____|____|____|____|____|____

Exercise: (Include Videos, Walking, Exercise equipment, Any type of exercise that you did)
After exercising I felt _____
Type_____ How Long: _____
Type_____ How Long: _____
Type_____ How Long: _____
Type_____ How Long: _____

Strength Training: After working out I felt:_____

_____X_____	Reps at _____	lbs
_____X_____	Reps at _____	lbs
_____X_____	Reps at _____	lbs
_____X_____	Reps at _____	lbs
_____X_____	Reps at _____	lbs
_____X_____	Reps at _____	lbs
_____X_____	Reps at _____	lbs
_____X_____	Reps at _____	lbs

Happiness involves working towards meaningful goals ~ Unknown Author

Today was: _____

I am on the right path ~ Melissa Alvarez

Daily Journal   Today's Date: _____   Weight: _____
My Mood: _____

Extra checklist boxes are to accommodate for various weight loss programs. You can check the boxes, list individual foods under Today Was page, keep a numerical log below or do all three.

Checklist: Bread/Starch: ☐☐☐☐☐☐☐☐, Protein: ☐☐☐☐☐☐☐☐
Veggies: ☐☐☐☐☐☐☐☐, Fruit: ☐☐☐☐☐☐☐☐, Fat: ☐☐☐☐☐,
Dairy: ☐☐☐☐☐☐☐, Water (8oz): ☐☐☐☐☐☐☐☐☐☐, Vitamin ☐

What I Ate: <u>Protein | Fat | Carbs| Fiber |Calories| Points | Other</u>

Breakfast: ____|____|____|____|____|____|____   Circle One
                                                                                Daily
Lunch: ____|____|____|____|____|____|____
                                                                                  ☺
Dinner: ____|____|____|____|____|____|____
                                                                                  😐
Snack: ____|____|____|____|____|____|____
                                                                                  ☹
Other Meal ____|____|____|____|____|____|____
                                                                                Hunger Level
Other Meal ____|____|____|____|____|____|____
                                                                                  +   −
Add it up: ____|____|____|____|____|____|____

Exercise: (Include Videos, Walking, Exercise equipment, Any type of exercise that you did)
After exercising I felt _____
Type_____ How Long: _____
Type_____ How Long: _____
Type_____ How Long: _____
Type_____ How Long: _____

Strength Training: After working out I felt:_____

_____	X_____	Reps at _____	lbs
_____	X_____	Reps at _____	lbs
_____	X_____	Reps at _____	lbs
_____	X_____	Reps at _____	lbs
_____	X_____	Reps at _____	lbs
_____	X_____	Reps at _____	lbs
_____	X_____	Reps at _____	lbs
_____	X_____	Reps at _____	lbs

I shall emerge as a new, revitalized person ~ Melissa Alvarez

Today was:

High expectations are the key to everything ~ Unknown Author

Daily Journal   Today's Date: _____   Weight: _____
My Mood: _____

Extra checklist boxes are to accommodate for various weight loss programs. You can check the boxes, list individual foods under Today Was page, keep a numerical log below or do all three.

Checklist: Bread/Starch: ☐☐☐☐☐☐☐☐, Protein: ☐☐☐☐☐☐☐☐
Veggies: ☐☐☐☐☐☐☐☐, Fruit: ☐☐☐☐☐☐☐☐, Fat: ☐☐☐☐☐,
Dairy: ☐☐☐☐☐☐☐, Water (8oz): ☐☐☐☐☐☐☐☐☐☐, Vitamin ☐

What I Ate: Protein | Fat | Carbs| Fiber |Calories| Points | Other

Breakfast: _____|_____|_____|_____|_____|_____|_____   Circle One
                                                              Daily
Lunch: _____|_____|_____|_____|_____|_____|_____
                                                               ☺
Dinner: _____|_____|_____|_____|_____|_____|_____
                                                               😐
Snack: _____|_____|_____|_____|_____|_____|_____
                                                               ☹
Other Meal _____|_____|_____|_____|_____|_____|_____
                                                          Hunger Level
Other Meal _____|_____|_____|_____|_____|_____|_____
                                                             +   -
Add it up: _____|_____|_____|_____|_____|_____|_____

Exercise: (Include Videos, Walking, Exercise equipment, Any type of exercise that you did)
After exercising I felt _____
Type_____ How Long: _____
Type_____ How Long: _____
Type_____ How Long: _____
Type_____ How Long: _____

Strength Training: After working out I felt:_____

_____ X_____ Reps at _____ lbs
_____ X_____ Reps at _____ lbs
_____ X_____ Reps at _____ lbs
_____ X_____ Reps at _____ lbs
_____ X_____ Reps at _____ lbs
_____ X_____ Reps at _____ lbs
_____ X_____ Reps at _____ lbs
_____ X_____ Reps at _____ lbs

The Phoenix's Guide To Self Renewal

If you don't know where you're going, you'll end up somewhere else ~ Unknown Author

Today was: _____

Improvement begins with "I" ~ Unknown Author

Daily Journal   Today's Date: _____   Weight: _____
My Mood: _____

Extra checklist boxes are to accommodate for various weight loss programs. You can check the boxes, list individual foods under Today Was page, keep a numerical log below or do all three.

Checklist: Bread/Starch: ☐☐☐☐☐☐☐☐, Protein: ☐☐☐☐☐☐☐☐
Veggies: ☐☐☐☐☐☐☐☐, Fruit: ☐☐☐☐☐☐☐☐, Fat: ☐☐☐☐☐,
Dairy: ☐☐☐☐☐☐☐, Water (8oz): ☐☐☐☐☐☐☐☐☐☐, Vitamin ☐

What I Ate: Protein | Fat | Carbs| Fiber |Calories| Points | Other

Breakfast: ____|____|____|____|____|____|____   Circle One
                                                      Daily
Lunch: ____|____|____|____|____|____|____
                                                       ☺
Dinner: ____|____|____|____|____|____|____
                                                       ☹
Snack: ____|____|____|____|____|____|____
                                                       ☹
Other Meal ____|____|____|____|____|____|____
                                                     Hunger Level
Other Meal ____|____|____|____|____|____|____
                                                       +   -
Add it up: ____|____|____|____|____|____|____

Exercise: (Include Videos, Walking, Exercise equipment, Any type of exercise that you did)
After exercising I felt _____
Type_____ How Long: _____
Type_____ How Long: _____
Type_____ How Long: _____
Type_____ How Long: _____

Strength Training: After working out I felt:_____

_____ X _____	Reps at	_____	lbs
_____ X _____	Reps at	_____	lbs
_____ X _____	Reps at	_____	lbs
_____ X _____	Reps at	_____	lbs
_____ X _____	Reps at	_____	lbs
_____ X _____	Reps at	_____	lbs
_____ X _____	Reps at	_____	lbs
_____ X _____	Reps at	_____	lbs

The secret of action is to begin ~ Unknown Author

Today was: _____

Make an effort everyday to feel good about who you are and what you can be ~
Unknown Author

Daily Journal   Today's Date: _____   Weight: _____
My Mood: _____

Extra checklist boxes are to accommodate for various weight loss programs. You can check the boxes, list individual foods under Today Was page, keep a numerical log below or do all three.

Checklist: Bread/Starch: ☐☐☐☐☐☐☐☐, Protein: ☐☐☐☐☐☐☐☐
Veggies: ☐☐☐☐☐☐☐☐, Fruit: ☐☐☐☐☐☐☐☐, Fat: ☐☐☐☐☐☐,
Dairy: ☐☐☐☐☐☐☐, Water (8oz): ☐☐☐☐☐☐☐☐☐☐, Vitamin ☐

What I Ate: Protein | Fat | Carbs| Fiber |Calories| Points | Other

Breakfast: ____|____|____|____|____|____|____

Lunch: ____|____|____|____|____|____|____

Dinner: ____|____|____|____|____|____|____

Snack: ____|____|____|____|____|____|____

Other Meal ____|____|____|____|____|____|____

Other Meal ____|____|____|____|____|____|____

Add it up: ____|____|____|____|____|____|____

Circle One
Daily

☺

☐ (neutral face)

☹

Hunger Level

+   −

Exercise: (Include Videos, Walking, Exercise equipment, Any type of exercise that you did)
After exercising I felt _____
Type_____ How Long: _____
Type_____ How Long: _____
Type_____ How Long: _____
Type_____ How Long: _____

Strength Training: After working out I felt:_____

_____ X _____	Reps at	_____ lbs
_____ X _____	Reps at	_____ lbs
_____ X _____	Reps at	_____ lbs
_____ X _____	Reps at	_____ lbs
_____ X _____	Reps at	_____ lbs
_____ X _____	Reps at	_____ lbs
_____ X _____	Reps at	_____ lbs
_____ X _____	Reps at	_____ lbs

I AM the Phoenix ~ Melissa Alvarez

Today was: _____

Knock the T off can't. You can if you think you can ~ Unknown Author

Daily Journal   Today's Date: _____   Weight: _____
My Mood: _____

Extra checklist boxes are to accommodate for various weight loss programs. You can check the boxes, list individual foods under Today Was page, keep a numerical log below or do all three.

Checklist: Bread/Starch: ☐☐☐☐☐☐☐☐, Protein: ☐☐☐☐☐☐☐☐
Veggies: ☐☐☐☐☐☐☐☐, Fruit: ☐☐☐☐☐☐☐☐, Fat: ☐☐☐☐☐,
Dairy: ☐☐☐☐☐☐☐☐, Water (8oz): ☐☐☐☐☐☐☐☐☐☐, Vitamin ☐

What I Ate: Protein | Fat | Carbs | Fiber | Calories | Points | Other

Breakfast: ____|____|____|____|____|____|____   Circle One Daily

Lunch: ____|____|____|____|____|____|____   ☺

Dinner: ____|____|____|____|____|____|____   😐

Snack: ____|____|____|____|____|____|____   ☹

Other Meal ____|____|____|____|____|____|____   Hunger Level

Other Meal ____|____|____|____|____|____|____   +   -

Add it up: ____|____|____|____|____|____|____

Exercise: (Include Videos, Walking, Exercise equipment, Any type of exercise that you did)
After exercising I felt _____
Type_____ How Long: _____
Type_____ How Long: _____
Type_____ How Long: _____
Type_____ How Long: _____

Strength Training: After working out I felt:_____

_____	X_____	Reps at _____	lbs
_____	X_____	Reps at _____	lbs
_____	X_____	Reps at _____	lbs
_____	X_____	Reps at _____	lbs
_____	X_____	Reps at _____	lbs
_____	X_____	Reps at _____	lbs
_____	X_____	Reps at _____	lbs
_____	X_____	Reps at _____	lbs

The Phoenix's Guide To Self Renewal

Never let a day go by without a dream ~ Unknown Author

Today was: _____

I will accept responsibility for my actions ~ Melissa Alvarez

Daily Journal   Today's Date: _____   Weight: _____
My Mood: _____

Extra checklist boxes are to accommodate for various weight loss programs. You can check the boxes, list individual foods under Today Was page, keep a numerical log below or do all three.

Checklist: Bread/Starch: ☐☐☐☐☐☐☐☐, Protein: ☐☐☐☐☐☐☐☐
Veggies: ☐☐☐☐☐☐☐☐ , Fruit: ☐☐☐☐☐☐☐☐, Fat: ☐☐☐☐☐☐,
Dairy: ☐☐☐☐☐☐☐, Water (8oz): ☐☐☐☐☐☐☐☐☐☐, Vitamin ☐

What I Ate: Protein | Fat | Carbs| Fiber |Calories| Points | Other

Breakfast: ____|____|____|____|____|____|____   Circle One Daily

Lunch: ____|____|____|____|____|____|____   ☺

Dinner: ____|____|____|____|____|____|____   😐

Snack: ____|____|____|____|____|____|____   ☹

Other Meal ____|____|____|____|____|____|____   Hunger Level

Other Meal ____|____|____|____|____|____|____   +   -

Add it up: ____|____|____|____|____|____|____

Exercise: (Include Videos, Walking, Exercise equipment, Any type of exercise that you did)
After exercising I felt _____
Type_____ How Long: _____
Type_____ How Long: _____
Type_____ How Long: _____
Type_____ How Long: _____

Strength Training: After working out I felt:_____

_____ X _____	Reps at _____	lbs
_____ X _____	Reps at _____	lbs
_____ X _____	Reps at _____	lbs
_____ X _____	Reps at _____	lbs
_____ X _____	Reps at _____	lbs
_____ X _____	Reps at _____	lbs
_____ X _____	Reps at _____	lbs
_____ X _____	Reps at _____	lbs

Give a little dream room to grow ~ Unknown Author

Today was:

Success is the proper utilization of failure ~Unknown Author

Daily Journal   Today's Date: _____   Weight: _____
My Mood: _____

Extra checklist boxes are to accommodate for various weight loss programs. You can check the boxes, list individual foods under Today Was page, keep a numerical log below or do all three.

Checklist: Bread/Starch: ☐☐☐☐☐☐☐☐, Protein: ☐☐☐☐☐☐☐
Veggies: ☐☐☐☐☐☐☐☐, Fruit: ☐☐☐☐☐☐☐☐, Fat: ☐☐☐☐☐,
Dairy: ☐☐☐☐☐☐☐, Water (8oz): ☐☐☐☐☐☐☐☐☐☐, Vitamin ☐

What I Ate: Protein | Fat | Carbs | Fiber | Calories | Points | Other

Breakfast: ____|____|____|____|____|____|____   Circle One Daily

Lunch: ____|____|____|____|____|____|____   ☺

Dinner: ____|____|____|____|____|____|____   😐

Snack: ____|____|____|____|____|____|____   ☹

Other Meal ____|____|____|____|____|____|____   Hunger Level

Other Meal ____|____|____|____|____|____|____   +   -

Add it up: ____|____|____|____|____|____|____

Exercise: (Include Videos, Walking, Exercise equipment, Any type of exercise that you did)
After exercising I felt _____
Type_____ How Long: _____
Type_____ How Long: _____
Type_____ How Long: _____
Type_____ How Long: _____

Strength Training: After working out I felt:_____

_____	X_____	Reps at _____	lbs
_____	X_____	Reps at _____	lbs
_____	X_____	Reps at _____	lbs
_____	X_____	Reps at _____	lbs
_____	X_____	Reps at _____	lbs
_____	X_____	Reps at _____	lbs
_____	X_____	Reps at _____	lbs
_____	X_____	Reps at _____	lbs

The spring in my step reflects the joy in my heart ~ Melissa Alvarez

Today was: _____

Remember when you were at your best? Now be there again ~ Unknown Author

Daily Journal   Today's Date: _____   Weight: _____
My Mood: _____

Extra checklist boxes are to accommodate for various weight loss programs. You can check the boxes, list individual foods under Today Was page, keep a numerical log below or do all three.

Checklist: Bread/Starch: ☐☐☐☐☐☐☐☐, **Protein:** ☐☐☐☐☐☐☐☐
Veggies: ☐☐☐☐☐☐☐☐, **Fruit:** ☐☐☐☐☐☐☐☐, **Fat:** ☐☐☐☐☐,
Dairy: ☐☐☐☐☐☐☐, **Water (8oz):** ☐☐☐☐☐☐☐☐☐☐, **Vitamin** ☐

What I Ate: Protein | Fat | Carbs| Fiber |Calories| Points | Other

Breakfast: __|__|__|__|__|__|__

Lunch: __|__|__|__|__|__|__

Dinner: __|__|__|__|__|__|__

Snack: __|__|__|__|__|__|__

Other Meal __|__|__|__|__|__|__

Other Meal __|__|__|__|__|__|__

Add it up: __|__|__|__|__|__|__

Circle One Daily

☺

😐

☹

Hunger Level

+   -

Exercise: (Include Videos, Walking, Exercise equipment, Any type of exercise that you did)
After exercising I felt _____
Type_____ How Long: _____
Type_____ How Long: _____
Type_____ How Long: _____
Type_____ How Long: _____

Strength Training: After working out I felt:_____

_____	X_____	Reps at _____	lbs
_____	X_____	Reps at _____	lbs
_____	X_____	Reps at _____	lbs
_____	X_____	Reps at _____	lbs
_____	X_____	Reps at _____	lbs
_____	X_____	Reps at _____	lbs
_____	X_____	Reps at _____	lbs
_____	X_____	Reps at _____	lbs

The Phoenix's Guide To Self Renewal

There's no elevator to success. You have to take the stairs ~ Unknown Author

Today was: _____

Use it or lose it ~ Unknown Author

Daily Journal   Today's Date: _____   Weight: _____
My Mood: _____

Extra checklist boxes are to accommodate for various weight loss programs. You can check the boxes, list individual foods under Today Was page, keep a numerical log below or do all three.

Checklist: Bread/Starch: ☐☐☐☐☐☐☐☐, Protein: ☐☐☐☐☐☐☐☐
Veggies: ☐☐☐☐☐☐☐☐, Fruit: ☐☐☐☐☐☐☐☐, Fat: ☐☐☐☐☐☐,
Dairy: ☐☐☐☐☐☐☐, Water (8oz): ☐☐☐☐☐☐☐☐☐☐, Vitamin ☐

What I Ate: Protein | Fat | Carbs | Fiber | Calories | Points | Other

Breakfast: ____|____|____|____|____|____|____

Lunch: ____|____|____|____|____|____|____

Dinner: ____|____|____|____|____|____|____

Snack: ____|____|____|____|____|____|____

Other Meal ____|____|____|____|____|____|____

Other Meal ____|____|____|____|____|____|____

Add it up: ____|____|____|____|____|____|____

Circle One
Daily

☺

😐

☹

Hunger Level

+ -

Exercise: (Include Videos, Walking, Exercise equipment, Any type of exercise that you did)
After exercising I felt _____
Type_____ How Long: _____
Type_____ How Long: _____
Type_____ How Long: _____
Type_____ How Long: _____

Strength Training: After working out I felt:_____

_____	X_____	Reps at	_____ lbs
_____	X_____	Reps at	_____ lbs
_____	X_____	Reps at	_____ lbs
_____	X_____	Reps at	_____ lbs
_____	X_____	Reps at	_____ lbs
_____	X_____	Reps at	_____ lbs
_____	X_____	Reps at	_____ lbs
_____	X_____	Reps at	_____ lbs

When things go wrong, don't go with them ~ Unknown Author

Today was:

Exercise, you don't have time not to ~ Unknown Author

Daily Journal Today's Date: _____   Weight: _____
My Mood: _____

Extra checklist boxes are to accommodate for various weight loss programs. You can check the boxes, list individual foods under Today Was page, keep a numerical log below or do all three.

Checklist: Bread/Starch: ☐☐☐☐☐☐☐☐, Protein: ☐☐☐☐☐☐☐☐
Veggies: ☐☐☐☐☐☐☐☐, Fruit: ☐☐☐☐☐☐☐☐, Fat: ☐☐☐☐☐☐,
Dairy: ☐☐☐☐☐☐☐☐, Water (8oz): ☐☐☐☐☐☐☐☐☐☐, Vitamin ☐

What I Ate: Protein | Fat | Carbs| Fiber |Calories| Points | Other

Breakfast: ____|____|____|____|____|____|____   Circle One
                                                     Daily
Lunch: ____|____|____|____|____|____|____
                                                        ☺
Dinner: ____|____|____|____|____|____|____
                                                        ☹
Snack: ____|____|____|____|____|____|____
                                                        ☹
Other Meal ____|____|____|____|____|____|____
                                                   Hunger Level
Other Meal ____|____|____|____|____|____|____
                                                      +   -
Add it up: ____|____|____|____|____|____|____

Exercise: (Include Videos, Walking, Exercise equipment, Any type of exercise that you did)
After exercising I felt _____
Type_____ How Long: _____
Type_____ How Long: _____
Type_____ How Long: _____
Type_____ How Long: _____

Strength Training: After working out I felt:_____

_____	X_____	Reps at _____	lbs
_____	X_____	Reps at _____	lbs
_____	X_____	Reps at _____	lbs
_____	X_____	Reps at _____	lbs
_____	X_____	Reps at _____	lbs
_____	X_____	Reps at _____	lbs
_____	X_____	Reps at _____	lbs
_____	X_____	Reps at _____	lbs

Ideas don't work unless you do ~ Unknown Author

Today was: _____

If you only look at what is, you might never attain what could be ~ Unknown Author

Daily Journal
Today's Date: _____ **Weight:** _____
My Mood: _____

Extra checklist boxes are to accommodate for various weight loss programs. You can check the boxes, list individual foods under Today Was page, keep a numerical log below or do all three.

Checklist: Bread/Starch: ☐☐☐☐☐☐☐☐, Protein: ☐☐☐☐☐☐☐☐
Veggies: ☐☐☐☐☐☐☐☐, Fruit: ☐☐☐☐☐☐☐☐, Fat: ☐☐☐☐☐,
Dairy: ☐☐☐☐☐☐☐, Water (8oz): ☐☐☐☐☐☐☐☐☐☐, Vitamin ☐

What I Ate: Protein | Fat | Carbs | Fiber | Calories | Points | Other

Breakfast: ___|___|___|___|___|___|___

Lunch: ___|___|___|___|___|___|___

Dinner: ___|___|___|___|___|___|___

Snack: ___|___|___|___|___|___|___

Other Meal ___|___|___|___|___|___|___

Other Meal ___|___|___|___|___|___|___

Add it up: ___|___|___|___|___|___|___

Circle One Daily

☺

☹

☹

Hunger Level

+   -

Exercise: (Include Videos, Walking, Exercise equipment, Any type of exercise that you did)
After exercising I felt _____
Type_____ How Long: _____
Type_____ How Long: _____
Type_____ How Long: _____
Type_____ How Long: _____

Strength Training: After working out I felt:_____

_____ X _____	Reps at _____	lbs
_____ X _____	Reps at _____	lbs
_____ X _____	Reps at _____	lbs
_____ X _____	Reps at _____	lbs
_____ X _____	Reps at _____	lbs
_____ X _____	Reps at _____	lbs
_____ X _____	Reps at _____	lbs
_____ X _____	Reps at _____	lbs

Think highly of yourself, for the world takes you at your own estimate ~
Unknown Author

Today was: _____

Sincerity gives wings to power ~ *Unknown Author*

Daily Journal   Today's Date: _____   Weight: _____
My Mood: _____

Extra checklist boxes are to accommodate for various weight loss programs. You can check the boxes, list individual foods under Today Was page, keep a numerical log below or do all three.

Checklist: Bread/Starch: ☐☐☐☐☐☐☐☐, Protein: ☐☐☐☐☐☐☐☐
Veggies: ☐☐☐☐☐☐☐☐, Fruit: ☐☐☐☐☐☐☐☐, Fat: ☐☐☐☐☐☐,
Dairy: ☐☐☐☐☐☐☐☐, Water (8oz): ☐☐☐☐☐☐☐☐☐☐, Vitamin ☐

What I Ate: Protein | Fat | Carbs | Fiber | Calories | Points | Other

Breakfast: ____|____|____|____|____|____|____   Circle One
                                                  Daily
Lunch: ____|____|____|____|____|____|____
                                                    ☺
Dinner: ____|____|____|____|____|____|____
                                                    ☹
Snack: ____|____|____|____|____|____|____
                                                    ☹
Other Meal ____|____|____|____|____|____|____
                                                  Hunger Level
Other Meal ____|____|____|____|____|____|____
                                                   +   -
Add it up: ____|____|____|____|____|____|____

Exercise: (Include Videos, Walking, Exercise equipment, Any type of exercise that you did)
After exercising I felt _____
Type_____ How Long: _____
Type_____ How Long: _____
Type_____ How Long: _____
Type_____ How Long: _____

Strength Training: After working out I felt:_____

_____	X_____	Reps at _____	lbs
_____	X_____	Reps at _____	lbs
_____	X_____	Reps at _____	lbs
_____	X_____	Reps at _____	lbs
_____	X_____	Reps at _____	lbs
_____	X_____	Reps at _____	lbs
_____	X_____	Reps at _____	lbs
_____	X_____	Reps at _____	lbs

If the truth be known, most successes are built on a multitude of failures ~
Unknown Author

Today was:

Make your own destiny, don't wait for it to come to you, life is not a rehearsal! ~
Unknown Author

Daily Journal   Today's Date: _____   Weight: _____
My Mood: _____

Extra checklist boxes are to accommodate for various weight loss programs. You can check the boxes, list individual foods under Today Was page, keep a numerical log below or do all three.

Checklist: Bread/Starch: ☐☐☐☐☐☐☐☐, Protein: ☐☐☐☐☐☐☐☐
Veggies: ☐☐☐☐☐☐☐☐, Fruit: ☐☐☐☐☐☐☐☐, Fat: ☐☐☐☐☐☐,
Dairy: ☐☐☐☐☐☐☐, Water (8oz): ☐☐☐☐☐☐☐☐☐☐, Vitamin ☐

What I Ate: Protein | Fat | Carbs| Fiber |Calories| Points | Other

Breakfast: ____|____|____|____|____|____|____

Lunch: ____|____|____|____|____|____|____

Dinner: ____|____|____|____|____|____|____

Snack: ____|____|____|____|____|____|____

Other Meal ____|____|____|____|____|____|____

Other Meal ____|____|____|____|____|____|____

Add it up: ____|____|____|____|____|____|____

Circle One
Daily

☺

😐

☹

Hunger Level

+   -

Exercise: (Include Videos, Walking, Exercise equipment, Any type of exercise that you did)
After exercising I felt _____
Type_____ How Long: _____
Type_____ How Long: _____
Type_____ How Long: _____
Type_____ How Long: _____

Strength Training: After working out I felt:_____

_____X_____	Reps at _____	lbs
_____X_____	Reps at _____	lbs
_____X_____	Reps at _____	lbs
_____X_____	Reps at _____	lbs
_____X_____	Reps at _____	lbs
_____X_____	Reps at _____	lbs
_____X_____	Reps at _____	lbs
_____X_____	Reps at _____	lbs

If you think positive, you can move a mountain in no time ~ Unknown Author

Today was: _____

Laughing helps. It's like jogging inside ~ Unknown Author

Daily Journal   Today's Date: _____   Weight: _____
My Mood: _____

Extra checklist boxes are to accommodate for various weight loss programs. You can check the boxes, list individual foods under Today Was page, keep a numerical log below or do all three.

Checklist: Bread/Starch: ☐☐☐☐☐☐☐☐, Protein: ☐☐☐☐☐☐☐☐
Veggies: ☐☐☐☐☐☐☐☐, Fruit: ☐☐☐☐☐☐☐☐, Fat: ☐☐☐☐☐☐,
Dairy: ☐☐☐☐☐☐☐, Water (8oz): ☐☐☐☐☐☐☐☐☐☐, Vitamin ☐

What I Ate: Protein | Fat | Carbs | Fiber | Calories | Points | Other

Breakfast: ____|____|____|____|____|____|____

Lunch: ____|____|____|____|____|____|____

Dinner: ____|____|____|____|____|____|____

Snack: ____|____|____|____|____|____|____

Other Meal ____|____|____|____|____|____|____

Other Meal ____|____|____|____|____|____|____

Add it up: ____|____|____|____|____|____|____

Circle One Daily

☺

😐

☹

Hunger Level

+   -

Exercise: (Include Videos, Walking, Exercise equipment, Any type of exercise that you did)
After exercising I felt _____
Type_____ How Long: _____
Type_____ How Long: _____
Type_____ How Long: _____
Type_____ How Long: _____

Strength Training: After working out I felt:_____

_____	X_____	Reps at _____ lbs
_____	X_____	Reps at _____ lbs
_____	X_____	Reps at _____ lbs
_____	X_____	Reps at _____ lbs
_____	X_____	Reps at _____ lbs
_____	X_____	Reps at _____ lbs
_____	X_____	Reps at _____ lbs
_____	X_____	Reps at _____ lbs

Anonymous kindness is powerful magic ~ Unknown Author

Today was: _____

Don't get lost in the fabric of your personal drama ~ Unknown Author

Daily Journal   Today's Date: _____   Weight: _____
My Mood: _____

Extra checklist boxes are to accommodate for various weight loss programs. You can check the boxes, list individual foods under Today Was page, keep a numerical log below or do all three.

Checklist: Bread/Starch: ☐☐☐☐☐☐☐☐, Protein: ☐☐☐☐☐☐☐☐
Veggies: ☐☐☐☐☐☐☐☐, Fruit: ☐☐☐☐☐☐☐☐, Fat: ☐☐☐☐☐☐,
Dairy: ☐☐☐☐☐☐☐☐, Water (8oz): ☐☐☐☐☐☐☐☐☐☐, Vitamin ☐

What I Ate: Protein | Fat | Carbs | Fiber | Calories | Points | Other

Breakfast: ____|____|____|____|____|____|____   Circle One
                                                                                   Daily
Lunch: ____|____|____|____|____|____|____
                                                                                    ☺
Dinner: ____|____|____|____|____|____|____
                                                                                    ☹
Snack: ____|____|____|____|____|____|____
                                                                                    ☹
Other Meal ____|____|____|____|____|____|____
                                                                           Hunger Level
Other Meal ____|____|____|____|____|____|____
                                                                                  + -
Add it up: ____|____|____|____|____|____|____

Exercise: (Include Videos, Walking, Exercise equipment, Any type of exercise that you did)
After exercising I felt _____
Type_____ How Long: _____
Type_____ How Long: _____
Type_____ How Long: _____
Type_____ How Long: _____

Strength Training: After working out I felt:_____

_____	X_____	Reps at _____	lbs
_____	X_____	Reps at _____	lbs
_____	X_____	Reps at _____	lbs
_____	X_____	Reps at _____	lbs
_____	X_____	Reps at _____	lbs
_____	X_____	Reps at _____	lbs
_____	X_____	Reps at _____	lbs
_____	X_____	Reps at _____	lbs

Humor prevents hardening of the attitudes ~ Unknown Author

Today was: _____

The Pessimist curses the wind...The Optimist hopes it will change...The Realist adjusts the sails ~ Unknown Author

Daily Journal   Today's Date: _____   Weight: _____
My Mood: _____

Extra checklist boxes are to accommodate for various weight loss programs. You can check the boxes, list individual foods under Today Was page, keep a numerical log below or do all three.

Checklist: Bread/Starch: ☐☐☐☐☐☐☐☐, Protein: ☐☐☐☐☐☐☐☐
Veggies: ☐☐☐☐☐☐☐☐, Fruit: ☐☐☐☐☐☐☐☐, Fat: ☐☐☐☐☐☐,
Dairy: ☐☐☐☐☐☐☐☐, Water (8oz): ☐☐☐☐☐☐☐☐☐☐, Vitamin ☐

What I Ate: <u>Protein | Fat | Carbs| Fiber |Calories| Points | Other</u>

Breakfast: ____|____|____|____|____|____|____   Circle One Daily

Lunch: ____|____|____|____|____|____|____   ☺

Dinner: ____|____|____|____|____|____|____   😐

Snack: ____|____|____|____|____|____|____   ☹

Other Meal ____|____|____|____|____|____|____
                                                    Hunger Level
Other Meal ____|____|____|____|____|____|____
                                                       +   -
Add it up: ____|____|____|____|____|____|____

Exercise: (Include Videos, Walking, Exercise equipment, Any type of exercise that you did)
After exercising I felt _____
Type_____ How Long: _____
Type_____ How Long: _____
Type_____ How Long: _____
Type_____ How Long: _____

Strength Training: After working out I felt:_____

_____X_____	Reps at	_____ lbs
_____X_____	Reps at	_____ lbs
_____X_____	Reps at	_____ lbs
_____X_____	Reps at	_____ lbs
_____X_____	Reps at	_____ lbs
_____X_____	Reps at	_____ lbs
_____X_____	Reps at	_____ lbs
_____X_____	Reps at	_____ lbs

I've learned - that we are responsible for what we do, no matter how we feel ~
Unknown Author

Today was:

If you want to go to the fruit of the tree...You have to go out on a limb ~
Unknown Author

Daily Journal   Today's Date: _____   Weight: _____
My Mood: _____

Extra checklist boxes are to accommodate for various weight loss programs. You can check the boxes, list individual foods under Today Was page, keep a numerical log below or do all three.

Checklist: Bread/Starch: ☐☐☐☐☐☐☐☐, Protein: ☐☐☐☐☐☐☐☐
Veggies: ☐☐☐☐☐☐☐☐, Fruit: ☐☐☐☐☐☐☐☐, Fat: ☐☐☐☐☐☐,
Dairy: ☐☐☐☐☐☐☐, Water (8oz): ☐☐☐☐☐☐☐☐☐☐, Vitamin ☐

What I Ate: Protein | Fat | Carbs | Fiber | Calories | Points | Other

Breakfast: ____|____|____|____|____|____|____

Lunch: ____|____|____|____|____|____|____

Dinner: ____|____|____|____|____|____|____

Snack: ____|____|____|____|____|____|____

Other Meal ____|____|____|____|____|____|____

Other Meal ____|____|____|____|____|____|____

Add it up: ____|____|____|____|____|____|____

Circle One
Daily

☺

☐

☹

Hunger Level

+   -

Exercise: (Include Videos, Walking, Exercise equipment, Any type of exercise that you did)
After exercising I felt _____
Type_____ How Long: _____
Type_____ How Long: _____
Type_____ How Long: _____
Type_____ How Long: _____

Strength Training: After working out I felt:_____

_____X_____	Reps at _____	lbs
_____X_____	Reps at _____	lbs
_____X_____	Reps at _____	lbs
_____X_____	Reps at _____	lbs
_____X_____	Reps at _____	lbs
_____X_____	Reps at _____	lbs
_____X_____	Reps at _____	lbs
_____X_____	Reps at _____	lbs

Obstacles are those frightful things you see when you take your eyes off your goals ~
Unknown Author

Today was: _____

The difference between ordinary and extraordinary is that little extra ~
Unknown Author

Daily Journal   Today's Date: _____   Weight: _____
My Mood: _____

Extra checklist boxes are to accommodate for various weight loss programs. You can check the boxes, list individual foods under Today Was page, keep a numerical log below or do all three.

Checklist: Bread/Starch: ☐☐☐☐☐☐☐☐, Protein: ☐☐☐☐☐☐☐☐
Veggies: ☐☐☐☐☐☐☐☐, Fruit: ☐☐☐☐☐☐☐☐, Fat: ☐☐☐☐☐,
Dairy: ☐☐☐☐☐☐☐, Water (8oz): ☐☐☐☐☐☐☐☐☐☐, Vitamin ☐

What I Ate: Protein | Fat | Carbs| Fiber |Calories| Points | Other

Breakfast: ____|____|____|____|____|____|____   Circle One
                                                    Daily
Lunch: ____|____|____|____|____|____|____
                                                    ☺
Dinner: ____|____|____|____|____|____|____
                                                    😐
Snack: ____|____|____|____|____|____|____
                                                    ☹
Other Meal ____|____|____|____|____|____|____
                                                    Hunger Level
Other Meal ____|____|____|____|____|____|____
                                                    +   -
Add it up: ____|____|____|____|____|____|____

Exercise: (Include Videos, Walking, Exercise equipment, Any type of exercise that you did)
After exercising I felt _____
Type_____ How Long: _____
Type_____ How Long: _____
Type_____ How Long: _____
Type_____ How Long: _____

Strength Training: After working out I felt:_____

_____ X _____ Reps at _____ lbs
_____ X _____ Reps at _____ lbs
_____ X _____ Reps at _____ lbs
_____ X _____ Reps at _____ lbs
_____ X _____ Reps at _____ lbs
_____ X _____ Reps at _____ lbs
_____ X _____ Reps at _____ lbs
_____ X _____ Reps at _____ lbs

Destiny is not a matter of chance, it is a matter of choice ~ Unknown Author

Today was: _____

Of all the things you wear, your expression is the most important ~ Unknown Author

Daily Journal   Today's Date: _____   Weight: _____
My Mood: _____

Extra checklist boxes are to accommodate for various weight loss programs. You can check the boxes, list individual foods under Today Was page, keep a numerical log below or do all three.

Checklist: Bread/Starch: ☐☐☐☐☐☐☐☐, Protein: ☐☐☐☐☐☐☐☐
Veggies: ☐☐☐☐☐☐☐☐, Fruit: ☐☐☐☐☐☐☐☐, Fat: ☐☐☐☐☐☐,
Dairy: ☐☐☐☐☐☐☐, Water (8oz): ☐☐☐☐☐☐☐☐☐☐, Vitamin ☐

What I Ate: Protein | Fat | Carbs| Fiber |Calories| Points | Other

Breakfast: ____|____|____|____|____|____|____

Lunch: ____|____|____|____|____|____|____

Dinner: ____|____|____|____|____|____|____

Snack: ____|____|____|____|____|____|____

Other Meal ____|____|____|____|____|____|____

Other Meal ____|____|____|____|____|____|____

Add it up: ____|____|____|____|____|____|____

Circle One
Daily

☺

☹

☹

Hunger Level

+   -

Exercise: (Include Videos, Walking, Exercise equipment, Any type of exercise that you did)
After exercising I felt _____
Type_____ How Long: _____
Type_____ How Long: _____
Type_____ How Long: _____
Type_____ How Long: _____

Strength Training: After working out I felt:_____

_____ X	_____	Reps at	____ lbs
_____ X	_____	Reps at	____ lbs
_____ X	_____	Reps at	____ lbs
_____ X	_____	Reps at	____ lbs
_____ X	_____	Reps at	____ lbs
_____ X	_____	Reps at	____ lbs
_____ X	_____	Reps at	____ lbs
_____ X	_____	Reps at	____ lbs

Learn from the mistakes of others. You can't live long enough to make them all yourself
~ Unknown Author

Today was: _____

Trust is the most valuable thing you will ever earn ~ Unknown Author

Daily Journal   Today's Date: _____   Weight: _____
My Mood: _____

Extra checklist boxes are to accommodate for various weight loss programs. You can check the boxes, list individual foods under Today Was page, keep a numerical log below or do all three.

Checklist: Bread/Starch: ☐☐☐☐☐☐☐☐, Protein: ☐☐☐☐☐☐☐☐
Veggies: ☐☐☐☐☐☐☐☐, Fruit: ☐☐☐☐☐☐☐☐, Fat: ☐☐☐☐☐☐,
Dairy: ☐☐☐☐☐☐☐, Water (8oz): ☐☐☐☐☐☐☐☐☐☐, Vitamin ☐

What I Ate: Protein | Fat | Carbs| Fiber |Calories| Points | Other

Breakfast: ____|____|____|____|____|____|____

Lunch: ____|____|____|____|____|____|____

Dinner: ____|____|____|____|____|____|____

Snack: ____|____|____|____|____|____|____

Other Meal ____|____|____|____|____|____|____

Other Meal ____|____|____|____|____|____|____

Add it up: ____|____|____|____|____|____|____

Circle One Daily

☺

☹

☹

Hunger Level

+ −

Exercise: (Include Videos, Walking, Exercise equipment, Any type of exercise that you did)
After exercising I felt _____
Type_____ How Long: _____
Type_____ How Long: _____
Type_____ How Long: _____
Type_____ How Long: _____

Strength Training: After working out I felt:_____

_____	X_____	Reps at _____	lbs
_____	X_____	Reps at _____	lbs
_____	X_____	Reps at _____	lbs
_____	X_____	Reps at _____	lbs
_____	X_____	Reps at _____	lbs
_____	X_____	Reps at _____	lbs
_____	X_____	Reps at _____	lbs
_____	X_____	Reps at _____	lbs

Each day comes bearing its gifts. Untie the ribbons ~ Unknown Author

Today was: _____

Laughter is the shock absorber that eases the blows of life ~ Unknown Author

Daily Journal   Today's Date: _____   Weight: _____
My Mood: _____

Extra checklist boxes are to accommodate for various weight loss programs. You can check the boxes, list individual foods under Today Was page, keep a numerical log below or do all three.

Checklist: Bread/Starch: ☐☐☐☐☐☐☐☐, Protein: ☐☐☐☐☐☐☐☐
Veggies: ☐☐☐☐☐☐☐☐, Fruit: ☐☐☐☐☐☐☐☐, Fat: ☐☐☐☐☐☐,
Dairy: ☐☐☐☐☐☐☐☐, Water (8oz): ☐☐☐☐☐☐☐☐☐☐, Vitamin ☐

What I Ate: Protein | Fat | Carbs| Fiber |Calories| Points | Other

Breakfast: ____|____|____|____|_____|_____|_____   Circle One
                                                            Daily
Lunch: ____|____|____|____|_____|_____|_____
                                                              ☺
Dinner: ____|____|____|____|_____|_____|_____
                                                              ☹
Snack: ____|____|____|____|_____|_____|_____
                                                              ☹
Other Meal ____|____|____|____|_____|_____|_____
                                                         Hunger Level
Other Meal ____|____|____|____|_____|_____|_____
                                                            +   -
Add it up: ____|____|____|____|_____|_____|_____

Exercise: (Include Videos, Walking, Exercise equipment, Any type of exercise that you did)
After exercising I felt _____
Type_____ How Long: _____
Type_____ How Long: _____
Type_____ How Long: _____
Type_____ How Long: _____

Strength Training: After working out I felt:_____

_____ X _____	Reps at	_____ lbs
_____ X _____	Reps at	_____ lbs
_____ X _____	Reps at	_____ lbs
_____ X _____	Reps at	_____ lbs
_____ X _____	Reps at	_____ lbs
_____ X _____	Reps at	_____ lbs
_____ X _____	Reps at	_____ lbs
_____ X _____	Reps at	_____ lbs

There is nothing about a caterpillar that tells you it's going to be a butterfly
~ *Unknown Author*

Today was: _____

Your ego can be an asset or a liability depending on how you relate to it ~
Unknown Author

Daily Journal   Today's Date: _____   Weight: _____
My Mood: _____

Extra checklist boxes are to accommodate for various weight loss programs. You can check the boxes, list individual foods under Today Was page, keep a numerical log below or do all three.

Checklist: Bread/Starch: ☐☐☐☐☐☐☐☐, Protein: ☐☐☐☐☐☐☐☐
Veggies: ☐☐☐☐☐☐☐☐, Fruit: ☐☐☐☐☐☐☐☐, Fat: ☐☐☐☐☐,
Dairy: ☐☐☐☐☐☐☐, Water (8oz): ☐☐☐☐☐☐☐☐☐☐, Vitamin ☐

What I Ate: Protein | Fat | Carbs| Fiber |Calories| Points | Other

Breakfast: ____|____|____|____|____|____|____

Lunch: ____|____|____|____|____|____|____

Dinner: ____|____|____|____|____|____|____

Snack: ____|____|____|____|____|____|____

Other Meal ____|____|____|____|____|____|____

Other Meal ____|____|____|____|____|____|____

Add it up: ____|____|____|____|____|____|____

Circle One
Daily

☺

☹

☹

Hunger Level

+   -

Exercise: (Include Videos, Walking, Exercise equipment, Any type of exercise that you did)
After exercising I felt _____
Type_____ How Long: _____
Type_____ How Long: _____
Type_____ How Long: _____
Type_____ How Long: _____

Strength Training: After working out I felt:_____

_____	X _____	Reps at _____	lbs
_____	X _____	Reps at _____	lbs
_____	X _____	Reps at _____	lbs
_____	X _____	Reps at _____	lbs
_____	X _____	Reps at _____	lbs
_____	X _____	Reps at _____	lbs
_____	X _____	Reps at _____	lbs
_____	X _____	Reps at _____	lbs

You will never get to where you want to be on dead hopes or hopeful wishing ~
Unknown Author

Today was: _____

Today is the yesterday you worried about tomorrow ~ Unknown Author

Daily Journal   Today's Date: _____   Weight: _____
My Mood: _____

Extra checklist boxes are to accommodate for various weight loss programs. You can check the boxes, list individual foods under Today Was page, keep a numerical log below or do all three.

Checklist: Bread/Starch: ☐☐☐☐☐☐☐☐, Protein: ☐☐☐☐☐☐☐☐
Veggies: ☐☐☐☐☐☐☐☐, Fruit: ☐☐☐☐☐☐☐☐, Fat: ☐☐☐☐☐,
Dairy: ☐☐☐☐☐☐☐, Water (8oz): ☐☐☐☐☐☐☐☐☐☐, Vitamin ☐

What I Ate: Protein | Fat | Carbs| Fiber |Calories| Points | Other

	Protein	Fat	Carbs	Fiber	Calories	Points	Other
Breakfast:							
Lunch:							
Dinner:							
Snack:							
Other Meal							
Other Meal							
Add it up:							

Circle One
Daily

☺

☹

☹

Hunger Level

\+   −

Exercise: (Include Videos, Walking, Exercise equipment, Any type of exercise that you did)
After exercising I felt _____
Type_____ How Long: _____
Type_____ How Long: _____
Type_____ How Long: _____
Type_____ How Long: _____

Strength Training: After working out I felt:_____

_____	X_____	Reps at _____	lbs
_____	X_____	Reps at _____	lbs
_____	X_____	Reps at _____	lbs
_____	X_____	Reps at _____	lbs
_____	X_____	Reps at _____	lbs
_____	X_____	Reps at _____	lbs
_____	X_____	Reps at _____	lbs
_____	X_____	Reps at _____	lbs

Drifting through life without aim or purpose is the first cause of failure ~
Unknown Author

Today was: _____

There is no failure. Only feedback. ~ Unknown Author

Daily Journal   Today's Date: _____   Weight: _____
My Mood: _____

Extra checklist boxes are to accommodate for various weight loss programs. You can check the boxes, list individual foods under Today Was page, keep a numerical log below or do all three.

Checklist: Bread/Starch: ☐☐☐☐☐☐☐☐☐, Protein: ☐☐☐☐☐☐☐☐
Veggies: ☐☐☐☐☐☐☐☐☐, Fruit: ☐☐☐☐☐☐☐☐, Fat: ☐☐☐☐☐☐,
Dairy: ☐☐☐☐☐☐☐☐, Water (8oz): ☐☐☐☐☐☐☐☐☐☐, Vitamin ☐

What I Ate: Protein | Fat | Carbs | Fiber | Calories | Points | Other

Breakfast:							
Lunch:							
Dinner:							
Snack:							
Other Meal							
Other Meal							
Add it up:							

Circle One
Daily

☺

😐

☹

Hunger Level

\+ −

Exercise: (Include Videos, Walking, Exercise equipment, Any type of exercise that you did)
After exercising I felt _____
Type_____ How Long: _____
Type_____ How Long: _____
Type_____ How Long: _____
Type_____ How Long: _____

Strength Training: After working out I felt:_____

_____	X_____	Reps at	_____ lbs
_____	X_____	Reps at	_____ lbs
_____	X_____	Reps at	_____ lbs
_____	X_____	Reps at	_____ lbs
_____	X_____	Reps at	_____ lbs
_____	X_____	Reps at	_____ lbs
_____	X_____	Reps at	_____ lbs
_____	X_____	Reps at	_____ lbs

Luck is when opportunity knocks and you answer ~ Unknown Author

Today was: _____

Happiness is like jam. You can't spread a little without getting some on yourself ~
Unknown Author

Daily Journal   Today's Date: _____   Weight: _____
My Mood: _____

Extra checklist boxes are to accommodate for various weight loss programs. You can check the boxes, list individual foods under Today Was page, keep a numerical log below or do all three.

Checklist: Bread/Starch: ☐ ☐ ☐ ☐ ☐ ☐ ☐ ☐, Protein: ☐ ☐ ☐ ☐ ☐ ☐ ☐ ☐
Veggies: ☐ ☐ ☐ ☐ ☐ ☐ ☐ ☐, Fruit: ☐ ☐ ☐ ☐ ☐ ☐ ☐ ☐, Fat: ☐ ☐ ☐ ☐ ☐ ☐,
Dairy: ☐ ☐ ☐ ☐ ☐ ☐ ☐, Water (8oz): ☐ ☐ ☐ ☐ ☐ ☐ ☐ ☐ ☐ ☐, Vitamin ☐

What I Ate: Protein | Fat | Carbs | Fiber | Calories | Points | Other

Breakfast: _____|_____|_____|_____|_____|_____|_____

Lunch: _____|_____|_____|_____|_____|_____|_____

Dinner: _____|_____|_____|_____|_____|_____|_____

Snack: _____|_____|_____|_____|_____|_____|_____

Other Meal _____|_____|_____|_____|_____|_____|_____

Other Meal _____|_____|_____|_____|_____|_____|_____

Add it up: _____|_____|_____|_____|_____|_____|_____

Circle One
Daily

☺

☹

☹

Hunger Level

\+ −

Exercise: (Include Videos, Walking, Exercise equipment, Any type of exercise that you did)
After exercising I felt _____
Type_____ How Long: _____
Type_____ How Long: _____
Type_____ How Long: _____
Type_____ How Long: _____

Strength Training: After working out I felt:_____

_____	X_____	Reps at _____	lbs
_____	X_____	Reps at _____	lbs
_____	X_____	Reps at _____	lbs
_____	X_____	Reps at _____	lbs
_____	X_____	Reps at _____	lbs
_____	X_____	Reps at _____	lbs
_____	X_____	Reps at _____	lbs
_____	X_____	Reps at _____	lbs

Seeing yourself as you want to be is the key to personal growth ~ Unknown Author

Today was: _____

We teach what we live ~ Unknown Author

Daily Journal
Today's Date: _____   Weight: _____
My Mood: _____

Extra checklist boxes are to accommodate for various weight loss programs. You can check the boxes, list individual foods under Today Was page, keep a numerical log below or do all three.

Checklist: Bread/Starch: ☐☐☐☐☐☐☐☐, Protein: ☐☐☐☐☐☐☐☐
Veggies: ☐☐☐☐☐☐☐☐, Fruit: ☐☐☐☐☐☐☐☐, Fat: ☐☐☐☐☐☐,
Dairy: ☐☐☐☐☐☐☐, Water (8oz): ☐☐☐☐☐☐☐☐☐☐, Vitamin ☐

What I Ate: <u>Protein | Fat | Carbs| Fiber |Calories| Points | Other</u>

Breakfast: ____|____|____|____|____|____|____

Lunch: ____|____|____|____|____|____|____

Dinner: ____|____|____|____|____|____|____

Snack: ____|____|____|____|____|____|____

Other Meal ____|____|____|____|____|____|____

Other Meal ____|____|____|____|____|____|____

Add it up: ____|____|____|____|____|____|____

Circle One Daily

☺

☹

☹

Hunger Level

\+   -

Exercise: (Include Videos, Walking, Exercise equipment, Any type of exercise that you did)
After exercising I felt _____
Type_____ How Long: _____
Type_____ How Long: _____
Type_____ How Long: _____
Type_____ How Long: _____

Strength Training: After working out I felt:_____

_____	X_____	Reps at _____	lbs
_____	X_____	Reps at _____	lbs
_____	X_____	Reps at _____	lbs
_____	X_____	Reps at _____	lbs
_____	X_____	Reps at _____	lbs
_____	X_____	Reps at _____	lbs
_____	X_____	Reps at _____	lbs
_____	X_____	Reps at _____	lbs

The meaning of life is to give life meaning ~ Unknown Author

Today was: _____

Faith is evidence of things unseen ~ Unknown Author

Daily Journal   Today's Date: _____   Weight: _____
My Mood: _____

Extra checklist boxes are to accommodate for various weight loss programs. You can check the boxes, list individual foods under Today Was page, keep a numerical log below or do all three.

Checklist: Bread/Starch: ☐☐☐☐☐☐☐☐, Protein: ☐☐☐☐☐☐☐☐
Veggies: ☐☐☐☐☐☐☐☐, Fruit: ☐☐☐☐☐☐☐☐, Fat: ☐☐☐☐☐,
Dairy: ☐☐☐☐☐☐☐, Water (8oz): ☐☐☐☐☐☐☐☐☐☐, Vitamin ☐

What I Ate: <u>Protein | Fat | Carbs| Fiber |Calories| Points | Other</u>

Breakfast:	___	___	___	___	___	___	___
Lunch:	___	___	___	___	___	___	___
Dinner:	___	___	___	___	___	___	___
Snack:	___	___	___	___	___	___	___
Other Meal	___	___	___	___	___	___	___
Other Meal	___	___	___	___	___	___	___
Add it up:	___	___	___	___	___	___	___

Circle One
Daily

☺

☹

☹

Hunger Level

+   -

Exercise: (Include Videos, Walking, Exercise equipment, Any type of exercise that you did)
After exercising I felt _____
Type_____ How Long: _____
Type_____ How Long: _____
Type_____ How Long: _____
Type_____ How Long: _____

Strength Training: After working out I felt:_____

_____ X _____	Reps at _____	lbs
_____ X _____	Reps at _____	lbs
_____ X _____	Reps at _____	lbs
_____ X _____	Reps at _____	lbs
_____ X _____	Reps at _____	lbs
_____ X _____	Reps at _____	lbs
_____ X _____	Reps at _____	lbs
_____ X _____	Reps at _____	lbs

If you can imagine it, you can achieve it, if you can dream it, you can become it ~
Unknown Author

Today was:

The love we give away is the only love we keep~ Unknown Author

Daily Journal   Today's Date: _____   Weight: _____
My Mood: _____

Extra checklist boxes are to accommodate for various weight loss programs. You can check the boxes, list individual foods under Today Was page, keep a numerical log below or do all three.

Checklist: Bread/Starch: ☐☐☐☐☐☐☐☐, Protein: ☐☐☐☐☐☐☐☐
Veggies: ☐☐☐☐☐☐☐☐, Fruit: ☐☐☐☐☐☐☐☐, Fat: ☐☐☐☐☐,
Dairy: ☐☐☐☐☐☐☐, Water (8oz): ☐☐☐☐☐☐☐☐☐☐, Vitamin ☐

What I Ate: Protein | Fat | Carbs | Fiber | Calories | Points | Other

Breakfast: ____|____|____|____|____|____|____   Circle One Daily

Lunch: ____|____|____|____|____|____|____   ☺

Dinner: ____|____|____|____|____|____|____   😐

Snack: ____|____|____|____|____|____|____   ☹

Other Meal ____|____|____|____|____|____|____
                                                     Hunger Level
Other Meal ____|____|____|____|____|____|____
                                                     +   -
Add it up: ____|____|____|____|____|____|____

Exercise: (Include Videos, Walking, Exercise equipment, Any type of exercise that you did)
After exercising I felt _____
Type_____ How Long: _____
Type_____ How Long: _____
Type_____ How Long: _____
Type_____ How Long: _____

Strength Training: After working out I felt:_____

_____	X _____	Reps at _____	lbs
_____	X _____	Reps at _____	lbs
_____	X _____	Reps at _____	lbs
_____	X _____	Reps at _____	lbs
_____	X _____	Reps at _____	lbs
_____	X _____	Reps at _____	lbs
_____	X _____	Reps at _____	lbs
_____	X _____	Reps at _____	lbs

He who knows others is wise. He who knows himself is enlightened~ Unknown Author

Today was:

The best way to predict your future is to create it. ~ *Unknown Author*

Daily Journal   Today's Date: _____   Weight: _____
My Mood: _____

Extra checklist boxes are to accommodate for various weight loss programs. You can check the boxes, list individual foods under Today Was page, keep a numerical log below or do all three.

Checklist: Bread/Starch: ☐☐☐☐☐☐☐☐, Protein: ☐☐☐☐☐☐☐☐
Veggies: ☐☐☐☐☐☐☐☐, Fruit: ☐☐☐☐☐☐☐☐, Fat: ☐☐☐☐☐,
Dairy: ☐☐☐☐☐☐☐, Water (8oz): ☐☐☐☐☐☐☐☐☐☐, Vitamin ☐

What I Ate: Protein | Fat | Carbs| Fiber |Calories| Points | Other

Breakfast: ____|____|____|____|____|____|____   Circle One
                                                  Daily
Lunch: ____|____|____|____|____|____|____
                                                  ☺
Dinner: ____|____|____|____|____|____|____
                                                  😐
Snack: ____|____|____|____|____|____|____
                                                  ☹
Other Meal ____|____|____|____|____|____|____
                                                  Hunger Level
Other Meal ____|____|____|____|____|____|____
                                                  +   −
Add it up: ____|____|____|____|____|____|____

Exercise: (Include Videos, Walking, Exercise equipment, Any type of exercise that you did)
After exercising I felt _____
Type_____ How Long: _____
Type_____ How Long: _____
Type_____ How Long: _____
Type_____ How Long: _____

Strength Training: After working out I felt:_____

_____ X_____	Reps at _____	lbs
_____ X_____	Reps at _____	lbs
_____ X_____	Reps at _____	lbs
_____ X_____	Reps at _____	lbs
_____ X_____	Reps at _____	lbs
_____ X_____	Reps at _____	lbs
_____ X_____	Reps at _____	lbs
_____ X_____	Reps at _____	lbs

You never really lose, until you quit trying ~ Unknown Author

Today was: _____

We should not let success go to our heads, or our failures go to our hearts~
Unknown Author

Daily Journal   Today's Date: _____   Weight: _____
My Mood: _____

Extra checklist boxes are to accommodate for various weight loss programs. You can check the boxes, list individual foods under Today Was page, keep a numerical log below or do all three.

Checklist: Bread/Starch: ☐☐☐☐☐☐☐☐, Protein: ☐☐☐☐☐☐☐☐
Veggies: ☐☐☐☐☐☐☐☐, Fruit: ☐☐☐☐☐☐☐☐, Fat: ☐☐☐☐☐☐,
Dairy: ☐☐☐☐☐☐☐, Water (8oz): ☐☐☐☐☐☐☐☐☐☐, Vitamin ☐

What I Ate: Protein | Fat | Carbs| Fiber |Calories| Points | Other

Breakfast: ____|____|____|____|____|____|____   Circle One Daily

Lunch: ____|____|____|____|____|____|____   ☺

Dinner: ____|____|____|____|____|____|____   😐

Snack: ____|____|____|____|____|____|____   ☹

Other Meal ____|____|____|____|____|____|____   Hunger Level

Other Meal ____|____|____|____|____|____|____   + -

Add it up: ____|____|____|____|____|____|____

Exercise: (Include Videos, Walking, Exercise equipment, Any type of exercise that you did)
After exercising I felt _____
Type_____ How Long: _____
Type_____ How Long: _____
Type_____ How Long: _____
Type_____ How Long: _____

Strength Training: After working out I felt:_____

_____ X _____	Reps at _____	lbs
_____ X _____	Reps at _____	lbs
_____ X _____	Reps at _____	lbs
_____ X _____	Reps at _____	lbs
_____ X _____	Reps at _____	lbs
_____ X _____	Reps at _____	lbs
_____ X _____	Reps at _____	lbs
_____ X _____	Reps at _____	lbs

A friend is one who believes in you when you have ceased to believe in yourself ~
Unknown Author

Today was:

The only thing in life achieved without effort is failure ~ Unknown Author

Daily Journal   Today's Date: _____   Weight: _____
My Mood: _____

Extra checklist boxes are to accommodate for various weight loss programs. You can check the boxes, list individual foods under Today Was page, keep a numerical log below or do all three.

Checklist: Bread/Starch: ☐☐☐☐☐☐☐☐, Protein: ☐☐☐☐☐☐☐☐
Veggies: ☐☐☐☐☐☐☐☐, Fruit: ☐☐☐☐☐☐☐☐, Fat: ☐☐☐☐☐☐,
Dairy: ☐☐☐☐☐☐☐☐, Water (8oz): ☐☐☐☐☐☐☐☐☐☐, Vitamin ☐

What I Ate: Protein | Fat | Carbs| Fiber |Calories| Points | Other

Breakfast: ____|____|____|____|____|____|____   Circle One
                                                            Daily
Lunch: ____|____|____|____|____|____|____
                                                             ☺
Dinner: ____|____|____|____|____|____|____
                                                             ☹
Snack: ____|____|____|____|____|____|____
                                                             ☹
Other Meal   ____|____|____|____|____|____|____
                                                          Hunger Level
Other Meal   ____|____|____|____|____|____|____
                                                            +   -
Add it up: ____|____|____|____|____|____|____

Exercise: (Include Videos, Walking, Exercise equipment, Any type of exercise that you did)
After exercising I felt _____
Type_____ How Long: _____
Type_____ How Long: _____
Type_____ How Long: _____
Type_____ How Long: _____

Strength Training: After working out I felt:_____

_____	X_____	Reps at _____	lbs
_____	X_____	Reps at _____	lbs
_____	X_____	Reps at _____	lbs
_____	X_____	Reps at _____	lbs
_____	X_____	Reps at _____	lbs
_____	X_____	Reps at _____	lbs
_____	X_____	Reps at _____	lbs
_____	X_____	Reps at _____	lbs

Anyone who says sunshine brings happiness has never danced in the rain ~
Unknown Author

Today was: _____

It's not who you are that holds you back, it's who you think you're not ~
Unknown Author

Daily Journal   Today's Date: _____   Weight: _____
My Mood: _____

Extra checklist boxes are to accommodate for various weight loss programs. You can check the boxes, list individual foods under Today Was page, keep a numerical log below or do all three.

Checklist: Bread/Starch: ☐ ☐ ☐ ☐ ☐ ☐ ☐ ☐, Protein: ☐ ☐ ☐ ☐ ☐ ☐ ☐ ☐
Veggies: ☐ ☐ ☐ ☐ ☐ ☐ ☐ ☐, Fruit: ☐ ☐ ☐ ☐ ☐ ☐ ☐ ☐, Fat: ☐ ☐ ☐ ☐ ☐ ☐,
Dairy: ☐ ☐ ☐ ☐ ☐ ☐ ☐, Water (8oz): ☐ ☐ ☐ ☐ ☐ ☐ ☐ ☐ ☐ ☐, Vitamin ☐

What I Ate: <u>Protein | Fat | Carbs| Fiber |Calories| Points | Other</u>

Breakfast: ____|____|____|____|____|____|____   Circle One Daily

Lunch: ____|____|____|____|____|____|____   ☺

Dinner: ____|____|____|____|____|____|____   ☐

Snack: ____|____|____|____|____|____|____   ☹

Other Meal ____|____|____|____|____|____|____   Hunger Level

Other Meal ____|____|____|____|____|____|____   + -

Add it up: ____|____|____|____|____|____|____

Exercise: (Include Videos, Walking, Exercise equipment, Any type of exercise that you did)
After exercising I felt _____
Type_____ How Long: _____
Type_____ How Long: _____
Type_____ How Long: _____
Type_____ How Long: _____

Strength Training: After working out I felt:_____

_____ X	_____	Reps at	_____ lbs
_____ X	_____	Reps at	_____ lbs
_____ X	_____	Reps at	_____ lbs
_____ X	_____	Reps at	_____ lbs
_____ X	_____	Reps at	_____ lbs
_____ X	_____	Reps at	_____ lbs
_____ X	_____	Reps at	_____ lbs
_____ X	_____	Reps at	_____ lbs

The Phoenix's Guide To Self Renewal

Let yourself get passionate about something~ Unknown Author

Today was: _____

Feel good about being a person who cares~ Unknown Author

Daily Journal   Today's Date: _____   Weight: _____
My Mood: _____

Extra checklist boxes are to accommodate for various weight loss programs. You can check the boxes, list individual foods under Today Was page, keep a numerical log below or do all three.

Checklist: Bread/Starch: ☐☐☐☐☐☐☐☐, Protein: ☐☐☐☐☐☐☐☐
Veggies: ☐☐☐☐☐☐☐☐, Fruit: ☐☐☐☐☐☐☐☐, Fat: ☐☐☐☐☐☐,
Dairy: ☐☐☐☐☐☐☐☐, Water (8oz): ☐☐☐☐☐☐☐☐☐☐, Vitamin ☐

What I Ate: Protein | Fat | Carbs| Fiber |Calories| Points | Other

Breakfast: ____|____|____|____|____|____|____   Circle One
                                                    Daily
Lunch: ____|____|____|____|____|____|____
                                                    ☺
Dinner: ____|____|____|____|____|____|____
                                                    😐
Snack: ____|____|____|____|____|____|____
                                                    ☹
Other Meal ____|____|____|____|____|____|____
                                                    Hunger Level
Other Meal ____|____|____|____|____|____|____
                                                    +   -
Add it up: ____|____|____|____|____|____|____

Exercise: (Include Videos, Walking, Exercise equipment, Any type of exercise that you did)
After exercising I felt _____
Type_____ How Long: _____
Type_____ How Long: _____
Type_____ How Long: _____
Type_____ How Long: _____

Strength Training: After working out I felt:_____

_____ X_____	Reps at _____	lbs
_____ X_____	Reps at _____	lbs
_____ X_____	Reps at _____	lbs
_____ X_____	Reps at _____	lbs
_____ X_____	Reps at _____	lbs
_____ X_____	Reps at _____	lbs
_____ X_____	Reps at _____	lbs
_____ X_____	Reps at _____	lbs

Live your dreams ~ Melissa Alvarez

Today was:

Joy can find you wherever you are ~ Unknown Author

Daily Journal   Today's Date: _____   Weight: _____
My Mood: _____

Extra checklist boxes are to accommodate for various weight loss programs. You can check the boxes, list individual foods under Today Was page, keep a numerical log below or do all three.

Checklist: Bread/Starch: ☐☐☐☐☐☐☐☐, Protein: ☐☐☐☐☐☐☐☐
Veggies: ☐☐☐☐☐☐☐☐, Fruit: ☐☐☐☐☐☐☐☐, Fat: ☐☐☐☐☐,
Dairy: ☐☐☐☐☐☐☐, Water (8oz): ☐☐☐☐☐☐☐☐☐☐, Vitamin ☐

What I Ate: Protein | Fat | Carbs | Fiber | Calories | Points | Other

	Protein	Fat	Carbs	Fiber	Calories	Points	Other
Breakfast:							
Lunch:							
Dinner:							
Snack:							
Other Meal							
Other Meal							
Add it up:							

Circle One Daily

☺
😐
☹

Hunger Level
+   −

Exercise: (Include Videos, Walking, Exercise equipment, Any type of exercise that you did)
After exercising I felt _____
Type_____ How Long: _____
Type_____ How Long: _____
Type_____ How Long: _____
Type_____ How Long: _____

Strength Training: After working out I felt:_____

_____	X _____	Reps at _____	lbs
_____	X _____	Reps at _____	lbs
_____	X _____	Reps at _____	lbs
_____	X _____	Reps at _____	lbs
_____	X _____	Reps at _____	lbs
_____	X _____	Reps at _____	lbs
_____	X _____	Reps at _____	lbs
_____	X _____	Reps at _____	lbs

You are a blessing that someone else counts ~ Unknown Author

Today was:

Think of today as a beautiful place you've never been ~ Unknown Author

Daily Journal   Today's Date: _____   Weight: _____
My Mood: _____

Extra checklist boxes are to accommodate for various weight loss programs. You can check the boxes, list individual foods under Today Was page, keep a numerical log below or do all three.

Checklist: Bread/Starch: ☐☐☐☐☐☐☐☐, Protein: ☐☐☐☐☐☐☐☐
Veggies: ☐☐☐☐☐☐☐☐, Fruit: ☐☐☐☐☐☐☐☐, Fat: ☐☐☐☐☐,
Dairy: ☐☐☐☐☐☐☐, Water (8oz): ☐☐☐☐☐☐☐☐☐☐, Vitamin ☐

What I Ate: Protein | Fat | Carbs | Fiber | Calories | Points | Other

Breakfast: ____|____|____|____|____|____|____

Lunch: ____|____|____|____|____|____|____

Dinner: ____|____|____|____|____|____|____

Snack: ____|____|____|____|____|____|____

Other Meal ____|____|____|____|____|____|____

Other Meal ____|____|____|____|____|____|____

Add it up: ____|____|____|____|____|____|____

Circle One Daily

☺

☹

☹

Hunger Level

\+ -

Exercise: (Include Videos, Walking, Exercise equipment, Any type of exercise that you did)
After exercising I felt _____
Type_____ How Long: _____
Type_____ How Long: _____
Type_____ How Long: _____
Type_____ How Long: _____

Strength Training: After working out I felt:_____

_____	X_____	Reps at _____	lbs
_____	X_____	Reps at _____	lbs
_____	X_____	Reps at _____	lbs
_____	X_____	Reps at _____	lbs
_____	X_____	Reps at _____	lbs
_____	X_____	Reps at _____	lbs
_____	X_____	Reps at _____	lbs
_____	X_____	Reps at _____	lbs

The poorest man is not without a cent but without a dream ~ Unknown Author

Today was: _____

I will not make excuses ~ Melissa Alvarez

Daily Journal   Today's Date: _____   Weight: _____
My Mood: _____

Extra checklist boxes are to accommodate for various weight loss programs. You can check the boxes, list individual foods under Today Was page, keep a numerical log below or do all three.

Checklist: Bread/Starch: ☐☐☐☐☐☐☐☐, Protein: ☐☐☐☐☐☐☐☐
Veggies: ☐☐☐☐☐☐☐☐, Fruit: ☐☐☐☐☐☐☐☐, Fat: ☐☐☐☐☐☐,
Dairy: ☐☐☐☐☐☐☐☐, Water (8oz): ☐☐☐☐☐☐☐☐☐☐, Vitamin ☐

What I Ate: Protein | Fat | Carbs | Fiber | Calories | Points | Other

Breakfast: _____|_____|_____|_____|_____|_____|_____   Circle One Daily

Lunch: _____|_____|_____|_____|_____|_____|_____   ☺

Dinner: _____|_____|_____|_____|_____|_____|_____   ☹

Snack: _____|_____|_____|_____|_____|_____|_____   ☹

Other Meal _____|_____|_____|_____|_____|_____|_____
                                                          Hunger Level
Other Meal _____|_____|_____|_____|_____|_____|_____
                                                          +   -
Add it up: _____|_____|_____|_____|_____|_____|_____

Exercise: (Include Videos, Walking, Exercise equipment, Any type of exercise that you did)
After exercising I felt _____
Type_____ How Long: _____
Type_____ How Long: _____
Type_____ How Long: _____
Type_____ How Long: _____

Strength Training: After working out I felt:_____

_____X_____	Reps at _____	lbs
_____X_____	Reps at _____	lbs
_____X_____	Reps at _____	lbs
_____X_____	Reps at _____	lbs
_____X_____	Reps at _____	lbs
_____X_____	Reps at _____	lbs
_____X_____	Reps at _____	lbs
_____X_____	Reps at _____	lbs

I am becoming healthier each and every day ~ Melissa Alvarez

Today was:

Great visions often start with small dreams ~ Unknown Author

Daily Journal   Today's Date: _____   Weight: _____
My Mood: _____

Extra checklist boxes are to accommodate for various weight loss programs. You can check the boxes, list individual foods under Today Was page, keep a numerical log below or do all three.

Checklist: Bread/Starch: ☐☐☐☐☐☐☐☐, Protein: ☐☐☐☐☐☐☐☐
Veggies: ☐☐☐☐☐☐☐☐, Fruit: ☐☐☐☐☐☐☐☐, Fat: ☐☐☐☐☐,
Dairy: ☐☐☐☐☐☐☐, Water (8oz): ☐☐☐☐☐☐☐☐☐☐, Vitamin ☐

What I Ate: Protein | Fat | Carbs| Fiber |Calories| Points | Other

Breakfast:	____	____	____	____	____	____	____
Lunch:	____	____	____	____	____	____	____
Dinner:	____	____	____	____	____	____	____
Snack:	____	____	____	____	____	____	____
Other Meal	____	____	____	____	____	____	____
Other Meal	____	____	____	____	____	____	____
Add it up:	____	____	____	____	____	____	____

Circle One
Daily

☺

☺

☹

Hunger Level

+   -

Exercise: (Include Videos, Walking, Exercise equipment, Any type of exercise that you did)
After exercising I felt _____
Type_____ How Long: _____
Type_____ How Long: _____
Type_____ How Long: _____
Type_____ How Long: _____

Strength Training: After working out I felt:_____

_____ X _____	Reps at _____	lbs
_____ X _____	Reps at _____	lbs
_____ X _____	Reps at _____	lbs
_____ X _____	Reps at _____	lbs
_____ X _____	Reps at _____	lbs
_____ X _____	Reps at _____	lbs
_____ X _____	Reps at _____	lbs
_____ X _____	Reps at _____	lbs

Habit is like a soft bed, easy to get into but hard to get out of ~ Unknown Author

Today was: _____

Let each day be your masterpiece ~ Unknown Author

Daily Journal Today's Date: _____ Weight: _____
My Mood: _____

Extra checklist boxes are to accommodate for various weight loss programs. You can check the boxes, list individual foods under Today Was page, keep a numerical log below or do all three.

Checklist: Bread/Starch: ☐☐☐☐☐☐☐☐, Protein: ☐☐☐☐☐☐☐☐
Veggies: ☐☐☐☐☐☐☐☐, Fruit: ☐☐☐☐☐☐☐☐, Fat: ☐☐☐☐☐☐,
Dairy: ☐☐☐☐☐☐☐, Water (8oz): ☐☐☐☐☐☐☐☐☐☐, Vitamin ☐

What I Ate: Protein | Fat | Carbs| Fiber |Calories| Points | Other

Breakfast:							
Lunch:							
Dinner:							
Snack:							
Other Meal							
Other Meal							
Add it up:							

Circle One
Daily

☺

☹

☹

Hunger Level
+ −

Exercise: (Include Videos, Walking, Exercise equipment, Any type of exercise that you did)
After exercising I felt _____
Type_____ How Long: _____
Type_____ How Long: _____
Type_____ How Long: _____
Type_____ How Long: _____

Strength Training: After working out I felt:_____

_____	X_____	Reps at	_____ lbs
_____	X_____	Reps at	_____ lbs
_____	X_____	Reps at	_____ lbs
_____	X_____	Reps at	_____ lbs
_____	X_____	Reps at	_____ lbs
_____	X_____	Reps at	_____ lbs
_____	X_____	Reps at	_____ lbs
_____	X_____	Reps at	_____ lbs

I believe in me! ~ Melissa Alvarez

Today was:

Forget mistakes. Organize victory out of mistakes ~ Unknown Author

Daily Journal   Today's Date: _____   Weight: _____
My Mood: _____

Extra checklist boxes are to accommodate for various weight loss programs. You can check the boxes, list individual foods under Today Was page, keep a numerical log below or do all three.

Checklist: Bread/Starch: ☐☐☐☐☐☐☐☐, Protein: ☐☐☐☐☐☐☐☐
Veggies: ☐☐☐☐☐☐☐☐, Fruit: ☐☐☐☐☐☐☐☐, Fat: ☐☐☐☐☐☐,
Dairy: ☐☐☐☐☐☐☐, Water (8oz): ☐☐☐☐☐☐☐☐☐☐, Vitamin ☐

What I Ate: <u>Protein | Fat | Carbs| Fiber |Calories| Points | Other</u>

Breakfast: ____|____|____|____|____|____|____   Circle One Daily

Lunch: ____|____|____|____|____|____|____

☺

Dinner: ____|____|____|____|____|____|____

😐

Snack: ____|____|____|____|____|____|____

☹

Other Meal ____|____|____|____|____|____|____

Hunger Level

Other Meal ____|____|____|____|____|____|____

+   -

Add it up: ____|____|____|____|____|____|____

Exercise: (Include Videos, Walking, Exercise equipment, Any type of exercise that you did)
After exercising I felt _____
Type_____ How Long: _____
Type_____ How Long: _____
Type_____ How Long: _____
Type_____ How Long: _____

Strength Training: After working out I felt:_____

_____	X_____	Reps at _____	lbs
_____	X_____	Reps at _____	lbs
_____	X_____	Reps at _____	lbs
_____	X_____	Reps at _____	lbs
_____	X_____	Reps at _____	lbs
_____	X_____	Reps at _____	lbs
_____	X_____	Reps at _____	lbs
_____	X_____	Reps at _____	lbs

I will be true to myself ~ Melissa Alvarez

Today was:

If you wait, all that happens is that you get older ~ Unknown Author

Daily Journal   Today's Date: _____   Weight: _____
My Mood: _____

Extra checklist boxes are to accommodate for various weight loss programs. You can check the boxes, list individual foods under Today Was page, keep a numerical log below or do all three.

Checklist: Bread/Starch: ☐☐☐☐☐☐☐☐, Protein: ☐☐☐☐☐☐☐☐
Veggies: ☐☐☐☐☐☐☐☐, Fruit: ☐☐☐☐☐☐☐☐, Fat: ☐☐☐☐☐☐,
Dairy: ☐☐☐☐☐☐☐, Water (8oz): ☐☐☐☐☐☐☐☐☐☐, Vitamin ☐

What I Ate: Protein | Fat | Carbs | Fiber | Calories | Points | Other

Breakfast: ____|____|____|____|____|____|____

Lunch: ____|____|____|____|____|____|____

Dinner: ____|____|____|____|____|____|____

Snack: ____|____|____|____|____|____|____

Other Meal ____|____|____|____|____|____|____

Other Meal ____|____|____|____|____|____|____

Add it up: ____|____|____|____|____|____|____

Circle One
Daily

☺

☹

☹

Hunger Level

\+   -

Exercise: (Include Videos, Walking, Exercise equipment, Any type of exercise that you did)
After exercising I felt _____
Type_____ How Long: _____
Type_____ How Long: _____
Type_____ How Long: _____
Type_____ How Long: _____

Strength Training: After working out I felt:_____

_____	X_____	Reps at _____	lbs
_____	X_____	Reps at _____	lbs
_____	X_____	Reps at _____	lbs
_____	X_____	Reps at _____	lbs
_____	X_____	Reps at _____	lbs
_____	X_____	Reps at _____	lbs
_____	X_____	Reps at _____	lbs
_____	X_____	Reps at _____	lbs

Nothing is hard if you try ~ Unknown Author

Today was:

Passion is the trigger of success ~ Unknown Author

Daily Journal   Today's Date: _____   Weight: _____
My Mood: _____

Extra checklist boxes are to accommodate for various weight loss programs. You can check the boxes, list individual foods under Today Was page, keep a numerical log below or do all three.

Checklist: Bread/Starch: ☐☐☐☐☐☐☐☐, Protein: ☐☐☐☐☐☐☐☐
Veggies: ☐☐☐☐☐☐☐☐, Fruit: ☐☐☐☐☐☐☐☐, Fat: ☐☐☐☐☐☐,
Dairy: ☐☐☐☐☐☐☐, Water (8oz): ☐☐☐☐☐☐☐☐☐☐, Vitamin ☐

What I Ate: Protein | Fat | Carbs| Fiber |Calories| Points | Other

Breakfast: ___|___|___|___|___|___|___   Circle One
                                              Daily
Lunch: ___|___|___|___|___|___|___
                                              ☺
Dinner: ___|___|___|___|___|___|___
                                              😐
Snack: ___|___|___|___|___|___|___
                                              ☹
Other Meal ___|___|___|___|___|___|___
                                              Hunger Level
Other Meal ___|___|___|___|___|___|___
                                              +   -
Add it up: ___|___|___|___|___|___|___

Exercise: (Include Videos, Walking, Exercise equipment, Any type of exercise that you did)
After exercising I felt _____
Type_____ How Long: _____
Type_____ How Long: _____
Type_____ How Long: _____
Type_____ How Long: _____

Strength Training: After working out I felt:_____

_____	X_____	Reps at _____ lbs
_____	X_____	Reps at _____ lbs
_____	X_____	Reps at _____ lbs
_____	X_____	Reps at _____ lbs
_____	X_____	Reps at _____ lbs
_____	X_____	Reps at _____ lbs
_____	X_____	Reps at _____ lbs
_____	X_____	Reps at _____ lbs

The more clear you are on what you want, the more power you will have ~
Unknown Author

Today was: _____

If it is to be, it is up to me ~ Unknown Author

Daily Journal   Today's Date: _____   Weight: _____
My Mood: _____

Extra checklist boxes are to accommodate for various weight loss programs. You can check the boxes, list individual foods under Today Was page, keep a numerical log below or do all three.

Checklist: Bread/Starch: ☐☐☐☐☐☐☐☐, Protein: ☐☐☐☐☐☐☐☐
Veggies: ☐☐☐☐☐☐☐☐, Fruit: ☐☐☐☐☐☐☐☐, Fat: ☐☐☐☐☐☐,
Dairy: ☐☐☐☐☐☐☐, Water (8oz): ☐☐☐☐☐☐☐☐☐☐, Vitamin ☐

What I Ate: Protein | Fat | Carbs| Fiber |Calories| Points | Other

Breakfast: _____|_____|_____|_____|_____|_____|_____

Lunch: _____|_____|_____|_____|_____|_____|_____

Dinner: _____|_____|_____|_____|_____|_____|_____

Snack: _____|_____|_____|_____|_____|_____|_____

Other Meal _____|_____|_____|_____|_____|_____|_____

Other Meal _____|_____|_____|_____|_____|_____|_____

Add it up: _____|_____|_____|_____|_____|_____|_____

Circle One Daily

☺

☻

☹

Hunger Level

+   -

Exercise: (Include Videos, Walking, Exercise equipment, Any type of exercise that you did)
After exercising I felt _____
Type_____ How Long: _____
Type_____ How Long: _____
Type_____ How Long: _____
Type_____ How Long: _____

Strength Training: After working out I felt:_____

_____ X _____	Reps at _____	lbs
_____ X _____	Reps at _____	lbs
_____ X _____	Reps at _____	lbs
_____ X _____	Reps at _____	lbs
_____ X _____	Reps at _____	lbs
_____ X _____	Reps at _____	lbs
_____ X _____	Reps at _____	lbs
_____ X _____	Reps at _____	lbs

Losers let it happen. Winners make it happen. ~ Unknown Author

Today was: _____

Morale is when your hand and feet keep on working when your head simply says it can't be done ~ Unknown Author

Daily Journal   Today's Date: _____ Weight: _____
My Mood: _____

Extra checklist boxes are to accommodate for various weight loss programs. You can check the boxes, list individual foods under Today Was page, keep a numerical log below or do all three.

Checklist: Bread/Starch: ☐☐☐☐☐☐☐☐, Protein: ☐☐☐☐☐☐☐☐
Veggies: ☐☐☐☐☐☐☐☐, Fruit: ☐☐☐☐☐☐☐☐, Fat: ☐☐☐☐☐☐,
Dairy: ☐☐☐☐☐☐☐☐, Water (8oz): ☐☐☐☐☐☐☐☐☐☐, Vitamin ☐

What I Ate: Protein | Fat | Carbs| Fiber |Calories| Points | Other

Breakfast: ____|____|____|____|____|____|____   Circle One Daily

Lunch: ____|____|____|____|____|____|____

☺

Dinner: ____|____|____|____|____|____|____

😐

Snack: ____|____|____|____|____|____|____

☹

Other Meal ____|____|____|____|____|____|____

Hunger Level

Other Meal ____|____|____|____|____|____|____

+   -

Add it up: ____|____|____|____|____|____|____

Exercise: (Include Videos, Walking, Exercise equipment, Any type of exercise that you did)
After exercising I felt _____
Type_____ How Long: _____
Type_____ How Long: _____
Type_____ How Long: _____
Type_____ How Long: _____

Strength Training: After working out I felt:_____

_____	X_____	Reps at _____	lbs
_____	X_____	Reps at _____	lbs
_____	X_____	Reps at _____	lbs
_____	X_____	Reps at _____	lbs
_____	X_____	Reps at _____	lbs
_____	X_____	Reps at _____	lbs
_____	X_____	Reps at _____	lbs
_____	X_____	Reps at _____	lbs

The best angle from which to approach any problem is the try-angle ~ *Unknown Author*

Today was: _____

The task ahead of us is never as great as the power behind us ~ Unknown Author

Daily Journal   Today's Date: _____   Weight: _____
My Mood: _____

Extra checklist boxes are to accommodate for various weight loss programs. You can check the boxes, list individual foods under Today Was page, keep a numerical log below or do all three.

Checklist: Bread/Starch: ☐☐☐☐☐☐☐☐, Protein: ☐☐☐☐☐☐☐☐
Veggies: ☐☐☐☐☐☐☐☐, Fruit: ☐☐☐☐☐☐☐☐, Fat: ☐☐☐☐☐,
Dairy: ☐☐☐☐☐☐☐☐, Water (8oz): ☐☐☐☐☐☐☐☐☐☐, Vitamin ☐

What I Ate: Protein | Fat | Carbs | Fiber | Calories | Points | Other

Breakfast: ____|____|____|____|____|____|____   Circle One Daily

Lunch: ____|____|____|____|____|____|____   ☺

Dinner: ____|____|____|____|____|____|____   😐

Snack: ____|____|____|____|____|____|____   ☹

Other Meal ____|____|____|____|____|____|____
                                                  Hunger Level
Other Meal ____|____|____|____|____|____|____
                                                  +   -
Add it up: ____|____|____|____|____|____|____

Exercise: (Include Videos, Walking, Exercise equipment, Any type of exercise that you did)
After exercising I felt _____
Type_____ How Long: _____
Type_____ How Long: _____
Type_____ How Long: _____
Type_____ How Long: _____

Strength Training: After working out I felt:_____

_____	X_____	Reps at _____	lbs
_____	X_____	Reps at _____	lbs
_____	X_____	Reps at _____	lbs
_____	X_____	Reps at _____	lbs
_____	X_____	Reps at _____	lbs
_____	X_____	Reps at _____	lbs
_____	X_____	Reps at _____	lbs
_____	X_____	Reps at _____	lbs

Most people are in favor of progress, it's the changes they don't like ~ Unknown Author

Today was:

Know yourself, master yourself, conquest of self is most gratifying ~ Unknown Author

Daily Journal
Today's Date: _____ **Weight:** _____
My Mood: _____

Extra checklist boxes are to accommodate for various weight loss programs. You can check the boxes, list individual foods under Today Was page, keep a numerical log below or do all three.

Checklist: Bread/Starch: ☐☐☐☐☐☐☐☐, Protein: ☐☐☐☐☐☐☐☐
Veggies: ☐☐☐☐☐☐☐☐, Fruit: ☐☐☐☐☐☐☐☐, Fat: ☐☐☐☐☐☐,
Dairy: ☐☐☐☐☐☐☐☐, Water (8oz): ☐☐☐☐☐☐☐☐☐☐, Vitamin ☐

What I Ate: Protein | Fat | Carbs | Fiber | Calories | Points | Other

Breakfast: ___|___|___|___|___|___|___

Lunch: ___|___|___|___|___|___|___

Dinner: ___|___|___|___|___|___|___

Snack: ___|___|___|___|___|___|___

Other Meal ___|___|___|___|___|___|___

Other Meal ___|___|___|___|___|___|___

Add it up: ___|___|___|___|___|___|___

Circle One
Daily

☺

☺

☹

Hunger Level

+   -

Exercise: (Include Videos, Walking, Exercise equipment, Any type of exercise that you did)
After exercising I felt _____
Type_____ How Long: _____
Type_____ How Long: _____
Type_____ How Long: _____
Type_____ How Long: _____

Strength Training: After working out I felt:_____

_____ X _____	Reps at _____	lbs
_____ X _____	Reps at _____	lbs
_____ X _____	Reps at _____	lbs
_____ X _____	Reps at _____	lbs
_____ X _____	Reps at _____	lbs
_____ X _____	Reps at _____	lbs
_____ X _____	Reps at _____	lbs
_____ X _____	Reps at _____	lbs

Passion burns in my soul, it is my desire that pushes me forward, and my unending persistence that enables me to attain my goals ~ Melissa Alvarez

Today was: _____

Take pride in how far you have come, have faith in how far you can go ~
Unknown Author

Daily Journal   Today's Date: _____   Weight: _____
My Mood: _____

Extra checklist boxes are to accommodate for various weight loss programs. You can check the boxes, list individual foods under Today Was page, keep a numerical log below or do all three.

Checklist: Bread/Starch: ☐ ☐ ☐ ☐ ☐ ☐ ☐ ☐, Protein: ☐ ☐ ☐ ☐ ☐ ☐ ☐ ☐
Veggies: ☐ ☐ ☐ ☐ ☐ ☐ ☐ ☐, Fruit: ☐ ☐ ☐ ☐ ☐ ☐ ☐ ☐, Fat: ☐ ☐ ☐ ☐ ☐ ☐,
Dairy: ☐ ☐ ☐ ☐ ☐ ☐ ☐ ☐, Water (8oz): ☐ ☐ ☐ ☐ ☐ ☐ ☐ ☐ ☐ ☐, Vitamin ☐

What I Ate: <u>Protein | Fat | Carbs| Fiber |Calories| Points | Other</u>

Breakfast: _____|_____|_____|_____|_____|_____|_____   Circle One
                                                                                              Daily
Lunch: _____|_____|_____|_____|_____|_____|_____
                                                                                                 ☺
Dinner: _____|_____|_____|_____|_____|_____|_____
                                                                                                 ☻
Snack: _____|_____|_____|_____|_____|_____|_____
                                                                                                 ☹
Other Meal _____|_____|_____|_____|_____|_____|_____
                                                                                            Hunger Level
Other Meal _____|_____|_____|_____|_____|_____|_____
                                                                                                +   -
Add it up: _____|_____|_____|_____|_____|_____|_____

Exercise: (Include Videos, Walking, Exercise equipment, Any type of exercise that you did)
After exercising I felt _____
Type_____ How Long: _____
Type_____ How Long: _____
Type_____ How Long: _____
Type_____ How Long: _____

Strength Training: After working out I felt:_____

_____ X _____	Reps at _____	lbs
_____ X _____	Reps at _____	lbs
_____ X _____	Reps at _____	lbs
_____ X _____	Reps at _____	lbs
_____ X _____	Reps at _____	lbs
_____ X _____	Reps at _____	lbs
_____ X _____	Reps at _____	lbs
_____ X _____	Reps at _____	lbs

Years wrinkle the skin, but lack of enthusiasm wrinkles the soul ~ Unknown Author

Today was: _____

Never let yesterday's disappointments overshadow tomorrow's dreams ~
Unknown Author

Daily Journal   Today's Date: _____   Weight: _____
My Mood: _____

Extra checklist boxes are to accommodate for various weight loss programs. You can check the boxes, list individual foods under Today Was page, keep a numerical log below or do all three.

Checklist: Bread/Starch: ☐☐☐☐☐☐☐☐, Protein: ☐☐☐☐☐☐☐☐
Veggies: ☐☐☐☐☐☐☐☐, Fruit: ☐☐☐☐☐☐☐☐, Fat: ☐☐☐☐☐☐,
Dairy: ☐☐☐☐☐☐☐, Water (8oz): ☐☐☐☐☐☐☐☐☐☐, Vitamin ☐

What I Ate: Protein | Fat | Carbs | Fiber | Calories | Points | Other

Breakfast: _____|_____|_____|_____|_____|_____|_____

Lunch: _____|_____|_____|_____|_____|_____|_____

Dinner: _____|_____|_____|_____|_____|_____|_____

Snack: _____|_____|_____|_____|_____|_____|_____

Other Meal _____|_____|_____|_____|_____|_____|_____

Other Meal _____|_____|_____|_____|_____|_____|_____

Add it up: _____|_____|_____|_____|_____|_____|_____

Circle One
Daily

☺

☹

☹

Hunger Level

+   -

Exercise: (Include Videos, Walking, Exercise equipment, Any type of exercise that you did)
After exercising I felt _____
Type_____ How Long: _____
Type_____ How Long: _____
Type_____ How Long: _____
Type_____ How Long: _____

Strength Training: After working out I felt:_____

_____ X _____	Reps at _____	lbs
_____ X _____	Reps at _____	lbs
_____ X _____	Reps at _____	lbs
_____ X _____	Reps at _____	lbs
_____ X _____	Reps at _____	lbs
_____ X _____	Reps at _____	lbs
_____ X _____	Reps at _____	lbs
_____ X _____	Reps at _____	lbs

Form good habits. They are just as hard to break as the bad ones! ~ Unknown Author

Today was: _____

The only consistency in life is change ~ Unknown Author

Daily Journal   Today's Date: _____   Weight: _____
My Mood: _____

Extra checklist boxes are to accommodate for various weight loss programs. You can check the boxes, list individual foods under Today Was page, keep a numerical log below or do all three.

Checklist: Bread/Starch: ☐ ☐ ☐ ☐ ☐ ☐ ☐ ☐, Protein: ☐ ☐ ☐ ☐ ☐ ☐ ☐ ☐
Veggies: ☐ ☐ ☐ ☐ ☐ ☐ ☐ ☐, Fruit: ☐ ☐ ☐ ☐ ☐ ☐ ☐ ☐, Fat: ☐ ☐ ☐ ☐ ☐ ☐,
Dairy: ☐ ☐ ☐ ☐ ☐ ☐ ☐ ☐, Water (8oz): ☐ ☐ ☐ ☐ ☐ ☐ ☐ ☐ ☐ ☐, Vitamin ☐

What I Ate: Protein | Fat | Carbs | Fiber | Calories | Points | Other

Breakfast: _____|_____|_____|_____|_____|_____|_____   Circle One
                                                                        Daily
Lunch: _____|_____|_____|_____|_____|_____|_____
                                                                           ☺
Dinner: _____|_____|_____|_____|_____|_____|_____
                                                                           ☹
Snack: _____|_____|_____|_____|_____|_____|_____
                                                                           ☹
Other Meal   _____|_____|_____|_____|_____|_____|_____
                                                                       Hunger Level
Other Meal   _____|_____|_____|_____|_____|_____|_____
                                                                          +   -
Add it up: _____|_____|_____|_____|_____|_____|_____

Exercise: (Include Videos, Walking, Exercise equipment, Any type of exercise that you did)
After exercising I felt _____
Type_____ How Long: _____
Type_____ How Long: _____
Type_____ How Long: _____
Type_____ How Long: _____

Strength Training: After working out I felt:_____

_____	X_____	Reps at _____	lbs
_____	X_____	Reps at _____	lbs
_____	X_____	Reps at _____	lbs
_____	X_____	Reps at _____	lbs
_____	X_____	Reps at _____	lbs
_____	X_____	Reps at _____	lbs
_____	X_____	Reps at _____	lbs
_____	X_____	Reps at _____	lbs

If I want circumstances in my life to change for the better, I must change for the better
~ *Unknown Author*

Today was: _____

Ideas are funny little things. They won't work unless you do ~ Unknown Author

Daily Journal   Today's Date: _____   Weight: _____
My Mood: _____

Extra checklist boxes are to accommodate for various weight loss programs. You can check the boxes, list individual foods under Today Was page, keep a numerical log below or do all three.

Checklist: Bread/Starch: ☐☐☐☐☐☐☐☐, Protein: ☐☐☐☐☐☐☐☐
Veggies: ☐☐☐☐☐☐☐☐, Fruit: ☐☐☐☐☐☐☐☐, Fat: ☐☐☐☐☐☐,
Dairy: ☐☐☐☐☐☐☐, Water (8oz): ☐☐☐☐☐☐☐☐☐☐, Vitamin ☐

What I Ate: Protein | Fat | Carbs | Fiber | Calories | Points | Other

Breakfast: ___|___|___|___|___|___|___

Lunch: ___|___|___|___|___|___|___

Dinner: ___|___|___|___|___|___|___

Snack: ___|___|___|___|___|___|___

Other Meal ___|___|___|___|___|___|___

Other Meal ___|___|___|___|___|___|___

Add it up: ___|___|___|___|___|___|___

Circle One
Daily

☺

☹

☹

Hunger Level

\+   -

Exercise: (Include Videos, Walking, Exercise equipment, Any type of exercise that you did)
After exercising I felt _____
Type_____ How Long: _____
Type_____ How Long: _____
Type_____ How Long: _____
Type_____ How Long: _____

Strength Training: After working out I felt:_____

_____ X _____	Reps at _____	lbs
_____ X _____	Reps at _____	lbs
_____ X _____	Reps at _____	lbs
_____ X _____	Reps at _____	lbs
_____ X _____	Reps at _____	lbs
_____ X _____	Reps at _____	lbs
_____ X _____	Reps at _____	lbs
_____ X _____	Reps at _____	lbs

Choose your actions carefully. What you do right now is creating the future in your world ~ Unknown Author

Today was: _____

A deadline has a marvelous ability to concentrate the mind ~ Unknown Author

Daily Journal   Today's Date: _____   Weight: _____
My Mood: _____

Extra checklist boxes are to accommodate for various weight loss programs. You can check the boxes, list individual foods under Today Was page, keep a numerical log below or do all three.

Checklist: Bread/Starch: ☐☐☐☐☐☐☐☐, Protein: ☐☐☐☐☐☐☐☐
Veggies: ☐☐☐☐☐☐☐☐, Fruit: ☐☐☐☐☐☐☐☐, Fat: ☐☐☐☐☐☐,
Dairy: ☐☐☐☐☐☐☐, Water (8oz): ☐☐☐☐☐☐☐☐☐☐, Vitamin ☐

What I Ate: Protein | Fat | Carbs| Fiber |Calories| Points | Other

Breakfast:							
Lunch:							
Dinner:							
Snack:							
Other Meal							
Other Meal							
Add it up:							

Circle One
Daily

☺

😐

☹

Hunger Level

\+   -

Exercise: (Include Videos, Walking, Exercise equipment, Any type of exercise that you did)
After exercising I felt _____
Type_____ How Long: _____
Type_____ How Long: _____
Type_____ How Long: _____
Type_____ How Long: _____

Strength Training: After working out I felt:_____

_____	X_____	Reps at _____	lbs
_____	X_____	Reps at _____	lbs
_____	X_____	Reps at _____	lbs
_____	X_____	Reps at _____	lbs
_____	X_____	Reps at _____	lbs
_____	X_____	Reps at _____	lbs
_____	X_____	Reps at _____	lbs
_____	X_____	Reps at _____	lbs

Triumph --umph added to try ~ Unknown Author

Today was: _____

All life is connected. When one part is damaged everything else is affected ~
Unknown Author

Daily Journal Today's Date: _____ Weight: _____
My Mood: _____

Extra checklist boxes are to accommodate for various weight loss programs. You can check the boxes, list individual foods under Today Was page, keep a numerical log below or do all three.

Checklist: Bread/Starch: ☐☐☐☐☐☐☐☐, Protein: ☐☐☐☐☐☐☐☐
Veggies: ☐☐☐☐☐☐☐☐, Fruit: ☐☐☐☐☐☐☐☐, Fat: ☐☐☐☐☐,
Dairy: ☐☐☐☐☐☐☐, Water (8oz): ☐☐☐☐☐☐☐☐☐☐, Vitamin ☐

What I Ate: Protein | Fat | Carbs | Fiber | Calories | Points | Other

Breakfast: _____|_____|_____|_____|_____|_____|_____   Circle One Daily

Lunch: _____|_____|_____|_____|_____|_____|_____   ☺

Dinner: _____|_____|_____|_____|_____|_____|_____   😐

Snack: _____|_____|_____|_____|_____|_____|_____   ☹

Other Meal _____|_____|_____|_____|_____|_____|_____
                                                                                        Hunger Level
Other Meal _____|_____|_____|_____|_____|_____|_____
                                                                                        +   -
Add it up: _____|_____|_____|_____|_____|_____|_____

Exercise: (Include Videos, Walking, Exercise equipment, Any type of exercise that you did)
After exercising I felt _____
Type_____ How Long: _____
Type_____ How Long: _____
Type_____ How Long: _____
Type_____ How Long: _____

Strength Training: After working out I felt:_____

_____ X _____	Reps at	_____	lbs
_____ X _____	Reps at	_____	lbs
_____ X _____	Reps at	_____	lbs
_____ X _____	Reps at	_____	lbs
_____ X _____	Reps at	_____	lbs
_____ X _____	Reps at	_____	lbs
_____ X _____	Reps at	_____	lbs
_____ X _____	Reps at	_____	lbs

If you don't hear opportunity knocking, find another door ~ Unknown Author

Today was: _____

The eyes are the window to the soul, as I look in the mirror I see myself as I truly am ~
Melissa Alvarez

Daily Journal   Today's Date: _____   Weight: _____
My Mood: _____

Extra checklist boxes are to accommodate for various weight loss programs. You can check the boxes, list individual foods under Today Was page, keep a numerical log below or do all three.

Checklist: Bread/Starch: ☐☐☐☐☐☐☐☐, Protein: ☐☐☐☐☐☐☐☐
Veggies: ☐☐☐☐☐☐☐☐, Fruit: ☐☐☐☐☐☐☐☐, Fat: ☐☐☐☐☐☐,
Dairy: ☐☐☐☐☐☐☐, Water (8oz): ☐☐☐☐☐☐☐☐☐☐, Vitamin ☐

What I Ate: Protein | Fat | Carbs | Fiber | Calories | Points | Other

Breakfast: ____|____|____|____|____|____|____

Lunch: ____|____|____|____|____|____|____

Dinner: ____|____|____|____|____|____|____

Snack: ____|____|____|____|____|____|____

Other Meal ____|____|____|____|____|____|____

Other Meal ____|____|____|____|____|____|____

Add it up: ____|____|____|____|____|____|____

Circle One Daily

☺

😐

☹

Hunger Level

\+   -

Exercise: (Include Videos, Walking, Exercise equipment, Any type of exercise that you did)
After exercising I felt _____
Type_____ How Long: _____
Type_____ How Long: _____
Type_____ How Long: _____
Type_____ How Long: _____

Strength Training: After working out I felt:_____

_____ X_____	Reps at _____	lbs
_____ X_____	Reps at _____	lbs
_____ X_____	Reps at _____	lbs
_____ X_____	Reps at _____	lbs
_____ X_____	Reps at _____	lbs
_____ X_____	Reps at _____	lbs
_____ X_____	Reps at _____	lbs
_____ X_____	Reps at _____	lbs

Keep your head and your heart going in the right direction and you will not have to worry about your feet ~ Unknown Author

Today was:

Seldom does an individual exceed his own expectations ~ Unknown Author

Daily Journal   Today's Date: _____   Weight: _____
My Mood: _____

Extra checklist boxes are to accommodate for various weight loss programs. You can check the boxes, list individual foods under Today Was page, keep a numerical log below or do all three.

Checklist: Bread/Starch: ☐☐☐☐☐☐☐☐, Protein: ☐☐☐☐☐☐☐☐
Veggies: ☐☐☐☐☐☐☐☐, Fruit: ☐☐☐☐☐☐☐☐, Fat: ☐☐☐☐☐,
Dairy: ☐☐☐☐☐☐☐, Water (8oz): ☐☐☐☐☐☐☐☐☐☐, Vitamin ☐

What I Ate: <u>Protein | Fat | Carbs| Fiber |Calories| Points | Other</u>

Breakfast: _____|_____|_____|_____|_____|_____|_____   Circle One Daily

Lunch: _____|_____|_____|_____|_____|_____|_____   ☺

Dinner: _____|_____|_____|_____|_____|_____|_____   😐

Snack: _____|_____|_____|_____|_____|_____|_____   ☹

Other Meal _____|_____|_____|_____|_____|_____|_____
                                                                 Hunger Level
Other Meal _____|_____|_____|_____|_____|_____|_____
                                                                    +   -
Add it up: _____|_____|_____|_____|_____|_____|_____

Exercise: (Include Videos, Walking, Exercise equipment, Any type of exercise that you did)
After exercising I felt _____
Type_____ How Long: _____
Type_____ How Long: _____
Type_____ How Long: _____
Type_____ How Long: _____

Strength Training: After working out I felt:_____

_____	X_____	Reps at _____ lbs
_____	X_____	Reps at _____ lbs
_____	X_____	Reps at _____ lbs
_____	X_____	Reps at _____ lbs
_____	X_____	Reps at _____ lbs
_____	X_____	Reps at _____ lbs
_____	X_____	Reps at _____ lbs
_____	X_____	Reps at _____ lbs

Reward yourself for all your hard work. You deserve it! ~ Unknown Author

Today was:

Minds are like parachutes...They only function when open ~ Unknown Author

Daily Journal   Today's Date: _____   Weight: _____
My Mood: _____

Extra checklist boxes are to accommodate for various weight loss programs. You can check the boxes, list individual foods under Today Was page, keep a numerical log below or do all three.

Checklist: Bread/Starch: ☐☐☐☐☐☐☐☐☐, Protein: ☐☐☐☐☐☐☐☐
Veggies: ☐☐☐☐☐☐☐☐☐, Fruit: ☐☐☐☐☐☐☐☐☐, Fat: ☐☐☐☐☐☐,
Dairy: ☐☐☐☐☐☐☐☐, Water (8oz): ☐☐☐☐☐☐☐☐☐☐, Vitamin ☐

What I Ate: Protein | Fat | Carbs | Fiber | Calories | Points | Other

Breakfast: ____|____|____|____|____|____|____

Lunch: ____|____|____|____|____|____|____

Dinner: ____|____|____|____|____|____|____

Snack: ____|____|____|____|____|____|____

Other Meal ____|____|____|____|____|____|____

Other Meal ____|____|____|____|____|____|____

Add it up: ____|____|____|____|____|____|____

Circle One
Daily

☺

☹

☹

Hunger Level

+   -

Exercise: (Include Videos, Walking, Exercise equipment, Any type of exercise that you did)
After exercising I felt _____
Type_____ How Long: _____
Type_____ How Long: _____
Type_____ How Long: _____
Type_____ How Long: _____

Strength Training: After working out I felt:_____

_____	X_____	Reps at ____	lbs
_____	X_____	Reps at ____	lbs
_____	X_____	Reps at ____	lbs
_____	X_____	Reps at ____	lbs
_____	X_____	Reps at ____	lbs
_____	X_____	Reps at ____	lbs
_____	X_____	Reps at ____	lbs
_____	X_____	Reps at ____	lbs

If you don't have time to do it right, you must have time to do it over ~
Unknown Author

Today was:

If nothing ever changed, there'd be no butterflies ~ Unknown Author

Daily Journal   Today's Date: _____   Weight: _____
My Mood: _____

Extra checklist boxes are to accommodate for various weight loss programs. You can check the boxes, list individual foods under Today Was page, keep a numerical log below or do all three.

Checklist: Bread/Starch: ☐☐☐☐☐☐☐☐, Protein: ☐☐☐☐☐☐☐☐
Veggies: ☐☐☐☐☐☐☐☐, Fruit: ☐☐☐☐☐☐☐☐, Fat: ☐☐☐☐☐,
Dairy: ☐☐☐☐☐☐☐, Water (8oz): ☐☐☐☐☐☐☐☐☐☐, Vitamin ☐

What I Ate: Protein | Fat | Carbs| Fiber |Calories| Points | Other

Breakfast: ____|____|____|____|____|____|____   Circle One
                                                    Daily
Lunch: ____|____|____|____|____|____|____
                                                     ☺
Dinner: ____|____|____|____|____|____|____
                                                     ☻
Snack: ____|____|____|____|____|____|____
                                                     ☹
Other Meal ____|____|____|____|____|____|____
                                                   Hunger Level
Other Meal ____|____|____|____|____|____|____
                                                     +   -
Add it up: ____|____|____|____|____|____|____

Exercise: (Include Videos, Walking, Exercise equipment, Any type of exercise that you did)
After exercising I felt _____
Type_____ How Long: _____
Type_____ How Long: _____
Type_____ How Long: _____
Type_____ How Long: _____

Strength Training: After working out I felt:_____

_____	X_____	Reps at _____	lbs
_____	X_____	Reps at _____	lbs
_____	X_____	Reps at _____	lbs
_____	X_____	Reps at _____	lbs
_____	X_____	Reps at _____	lbs
_____	X_____	Reps at _____	lbs
_____	X_____	Reps at _____	lbs
_____	X_____	Reps at _____	lbs

Behold the turtle; he only goes forward when his neck is stuck out ~ Unknown Author

Today was:

Yin and Yang: A blend of opposites for perfect harmony ~ Unknown Author

Daily Journal   Today's Date: _____   Weight: _____
My Mood: _____

Extra checklist boxes are to accommodate for various weight loss programs. You can check the boxes, list individual foods under Today Was page, keep a numerical log below or do all three.

Checklist: Bread/Starch: ☐☐☐☐☐☐☐☐, Protein: ☐☐☐☐☐☐☐☐
Veggies: ☐☐☐☐☐☐☐☐, Fruit: ☐☐☐☐☐☐☐☐, Fat: ☐☐☐☐☐,
Dairy: ☐☐☐☐☐☐☐, Water (8oz): ☐☐☐☐☐☐☐☐☐☐, Vitamin ☐

What I Ate: Protein | Fat | Carbs | Fiber | Calories | Points | Other

Breakfast: ____|____|____|____|____|____|____   Circle One
                                                   Daily
Lunch: ____|____|____|____|____|____|____
                                                   ☺
Dinner: ____|____|____|____|____|____|____
                                                   😐
Snack: ____|____|____|____|____|____|____
                                                   ☹
Other Meal ____|____|____|____|____|____|____
                                                   Hunger Level
Other Meal ____|____|____|____|____|____|____
                                                   +   -
Add it up: ____|____|____|____|____|____|____

Exercise: (Include Videos, Walking, Exercise equipment, Any type of exercise that you did)
After exercising I felt _____
Type_____ How Long: _____
Type_____ How Long: _____
Type_____ How Long: _____
Type_____ How Long: _____

Strength Training: After working out I felt: _____

_____	X_____	Reps at _____	lbs
_____	X_____	Reps at _____	lbs
_____	X_____	Reps at _____	lbs
_____	X_____	Reps at _____	lbs
_____	X_____	Reps at _____	lbs
_____	X_____	Reps at _____	lbs
_____	X_____	Reps at _____	lbs
_____	X_____	Reps at _____	lbs

We can do anything we want if we stick to it long enough ~ Unknown Author

Today was: _____

Failure is the path of least persistence ~ Unknown Author

Daily Journal   Today's Date: _____   Weight: _____
My Mood: _____

Extra checklist boxes are to accommodate for various weight loss programs. You can check the boxes, list individual foods under Today Was page, keep a numerical log below or do all three.

Checklist: Bread/Starch: ☐☐☐☐☐☐☐☐, Protein: ☐☐☐☐☐☐☐☐
Veggies: ☐☐☐☐☐☐☐☐, Fruit: ☐☐☐☐☐☐☐☐, Fat: ☐☐☐☐☐☐,
Dairy: ☐☐☐☐☐☐☐, Water (8oz): ☐☐☐☐☐☐☐☐☐☐, Vitamin ☐

What I Ate: Protein | Fat | Carbs| Fiber |Calories| Points | Other

	Protein	Fat	Carbs	Fiber	Calories	Points	Other
Breakfast:							
Lunch:							
Dinner:							
Snack:							
Other Meal							
Other Meal							
Add it up:							

Circle One
Daily

☺

☹

☚

Hunger Level

+   -

Exercise: (Include Videos, Walking, Exercise equipment, Any type of exercise that you did)
After exercising I felt _____
Type_____ How Long: _____
Type_____ How Long: _____
Type_____ How Long: _____
Type_____ How Long: _____

Strength Training: After working out I felt:_____

_____	X_____	Reps at _____	lbs
_____	X_____	Reps at _____	lbs
_____	X_____	Reps at _____	lbs
_____	X_____	Reps at _____	lbs
_____	X_____	Reps at _____	lbs
_____	X_____	Reps at _____	lbs
_____	X_____	Reps at _____	lbs
_____	X_____	Reps at _____	lbs

Winners know that accomplishment is the result of activity ~ Unknown Author

Today was:

Every accomplishment starts with the decision to try ~ Unknown Author

Daily Journal   Today's Date: _____   Weight: _____
My Mood: _____

Extra checklist boxes are to accommodate for various weight loss programs. You can check the boxes, list individual foods under Today Was page, keep a numerical log below or do all three.

Checklist: Bread/Starch: ☐☐☐☐☐☐☐☐, Protein: ☐☐☐☐☐☐☐☐
Veggies: ☐☐☐☐☐☐☐☐, Fruit: ☐☐☐☐☐☐☐☐, Fat: ☐☐☐☐☐,
Dairy: ☐☐☐☐☐☐☐, Water (8oz): ☐☐☐☐☐☐☐☐☐☐, Vitamin ☐

What I Ate: Protein | Fat | Carbs| Fiber |Calories| Points | Other

Breakfast: ____|____|____|____|____|____|____

Lunch: ____|____|____|____|____|____|____

Dinner: ____|____|____|____|____|____|____

Snack: ____|____|____|____|____|____|____

Other Meal ____|____|____|____|____|____|____

Other Meal ____|____|____|____|____|____|____

Add it up: ____|____|____|____|____|____|____

Circle One Daily

☺

☐

☹

Hunger Level

+   -

Exercise: (Include Videos, Walking, Exercise equipment, Any type of exercise that you did)
After exercising I felt _____
Type_____ How Long: _____
Type_____ How Long: _____
Type_____ How Long: _____
Type_____ How Long: _____

Strength Training: After working out I felt: _____

_____ X _____	Reps at _____	lbs
_____ X _____	Reps at _____	lbs
_____ X _____	Reps at _____	lbs
_____ X _____	Reps at _____	lbs
_____ X _____	Reps at _____	lbs
_____ X _____	Reps at _____	lbs
_____ X _____	Reps at _____	lbs
_____ X _____	Reps at _____	lbs

The dictionary is the only place that success comes before work. ~ Unknown Author

Today was: _____

It doesn't matter what you can do, what matters is what you will do ~
Unknown Author

Daily Journal

Today's Date: _____   Weight: _____

My Mood: _____

Extra checklist boxes are to accommodate for various weight loss programs. You can check the boxes, list individual foods under Today Was page, keep a numerical log below or do all three.

Checklist: Bread/Starch: ☐☐☐☐☐☐☐☐, Protein: ☐☐☐☐☐☐☐☐
Veggies: ☐☐☐☐☐☐☐☐, Fruit: ☐☐☐☐☐☐☐☐, Fat: ☐☐☐☐☐☐,
Dairy: ☐☐☐☐☐☐☐☐, Water (8oz): ☐☐☐☐☐☐☐☐☐☐, Vitamin ☐

What I Ate: Protein | Fat | Carbs | Fiber | Calories | Points | Other

Breakfast: _____|_____|_____|_____|_____|_____|_____   Circle One
                                                                    Daily
Lunch: _____|_____|_____|_____|_____|_____|_____
                                                                      ☺
Dinner: _____|_____|_____|_____|_____|_____|_____
                                                                      😐
Snack: _____|_____|_____|_____|_____|_____|_____
                                                                      ☹
Other Meal _____|_____|_____|_____|_____|_____|_____
                                                                 Hunger Level
Other Meal _____|_____|_____|_____|_____|_____|_____
                                                                    +   -
Add it up: _____|_____|_____|_____|_____|_____|_____

Exercise: (Include Videos, Walking, Exercise equipment, Any type of exercise that you did)
After exercising I felt _____
Type_____ How Long: _____
Type_____ How Long: _____
Type_____ How Long: _____
Type_____ How Long: _____

Strength Training: After working out I felt:_____

_____X_____	Reps at _____	lbs
_____X_____	Reps at _____	lbs
_____X_____	Reps at _____	lbs
_____X_____	Reps at _____	lbs
_____X_____	Reps at _____	lbs
_____X_____	Reps at _____	lbs
_____X_____	Reps at _____	lbs
_____X_____	Reps at _____	lbs

Don't just exist, LIVE ~ Unknown Author

Today was:

Champions believe in themselves even if no one else does ~ Unknown Author

Daily Journal   Today's Date: _____   Weight: _____
My Mood: _____

Extra checklist boxes are to accommodate for various weight loss programs. You can check the boxes, list individual foods under Today Was page, keep a numerical log below or do all three.

Checklist: Bread/Starch: ☐ ☐ ☐ ☐ ☐ ☐ ☐ ☐, Protein: ☐ ☐ ☐ ☐ ☐ ☐ ☐ ☐
Veggies: ☐ ☐ ☐ ☐ ☐ ☐ ☐ ☐, Fruit: ☐ ☐ ☐ ☐ ☐ ☐ ☐ ☐, Fat: ☐ ☐ ☐ ☐ ☐,
Dairy: ☐ ☐ ☐ ☐ ☐ ☐ ☐, Water (8oz): ☐ ☐ ☐ ☐ ☐ ☐ ☐ ☐ ☐ ☐, Vitamin ☐

What I Ate: Protein | Fat | Carbs| Fiber |Calories| Points | Other

Breakfast: ____|____|____|____|____|____|____   Circle One
                                                        Daily
Lunch: ____|____|____|____|____|____|____
                                                         ☺
Dinner: ____|____|____|____|____|____|____
                                                         ☹
Snack: ____|____|____|____|____|____|____
                                                         ☹
Other Meal ____|____|____|____|____|____|____
                                                       Hunger Level
Other Meal ____|____|____|____|____|____|____
                                                          +   -
Add it up: ____|____|____|____|____|____|____

Exercise: (Include Videos, Walking, Exercise equipment, Any type of exercise that you did)
After exercising I felt _____
Type_____ How Long: _____
Type_____ How Long: _____
Type_____ How Long: _____
Type_____ How Long: _____

Strength Training: After working out I felt:_____

_____X_____	Reps at _____	lbs
_____X_____	Reps at _____	lbs
_____X_____	Reps at _____	lbs
_____X_____	Reps at _____	lbs
_____X_____	Reps at _____	lbs
_____X_____	Reps at _____	lbs
_____X_____	Reps at _____	lbs
_____X_____	Reps at _____	lbs

Impossibility is an opinion, not a fact ~ Unknown Author

Today was: _____

Procrastination is the natural assassin of opportunity ~ Unknown Author

Daily Journal   Today's Date: _____   Weight: _____
My Mood: _____

Extra checklist boxes are to accommodate for various weight loss programs. You can check the boxes, list individual foods under Today Was page, keep a numerical log below or do all three.

Checklist: Bread/Starch: ☐ ☐ ☐ ☐ ☐ ☐ ☐ ☐, Protein: ☐ ☐ ☐ ☐ ☐ ☐ ☐ ☐
Veggies: ☐ ☐ ☐ ☐ ☐ ☐ ☐ ☐, Fruit: ☐ ☐ ☐ ☐ ☐ ☐ ☐ ☐, Fat: ☐ ☐ ☐ ☐ ☐,
Dairy: ☐ ☐ ☐ ☐ ☐ ☐ ☐, Water (8oz): ☐ ☐ ☐ ☐ ☐ ☐ ☐ ☐ ☐ ☐, Vitamin ☐

What I Ate: Protein | Fat | Carbs | Fiber | Calories | Points | Other

Breakfast:							
Lunch:							
Dinner:							
Snack:							
Other Meal							
Other Meal							
Add it up:							

Circle One
Daily

☺

😐

☹

Hunger Level

+   −

Exercise: (Include Videos, Walking, Exercise equipment, Any type of exercise that you did)
After exercising I felt _____
Type_____ How Long: _____
Type_____ How Long: _____
Type_____ How Long: _____
Type_____ How Long: _____

Strength Training: After working out I felt:_____

_____	X_____	Reps at ____	lbs
_____	X_____	Reps at ____	lbs
_____	X_____	Reps at ____	lbs
_____	X_____	Reps at ____	lbs
_____	X_____	Reps at ____	lbs
_____	X_____	Reps at ____	lbs
_____	X_____	Reps at ____	lbs
_____	X_____	Reps at ____	lbs

You've only failed, If you've failed to try ~ Unknown Author

Today was: _____

A smile is contagious - start an epidemic! ~ *Unknown Author*

Daily Journal Today's Date: _____ Weight: _____
My Mood: _____

Extra checklist boxes are to accommodate for various weight loss programs. You can check the boxes, list individual foods under Today Was page, keep a numerical log below or do all three.

Checklist: Bread/Starch: ☐☐☐☐☐☐☐☐, Protein: ☐☐☐☐☐☐☐☐
Veggies: ☐☐☐☐☐☐☐☐, Fruit: ☐☐☐☐☐☐☐☐, Fat: ☐☐☐☐☐☐,
Dairy: ☐☐☐☐☐☐☐, Water (8oz): ☐☐☐☐☐☐☐☐☐☐, Vitamin ☐

What I Ate: Protein | Fat | Carbs | Fiber | Calories | Points | Other

	Protein	Fat	Carbs	Fiber	Calories	Points	Other
Breakfast:							
Lunch:							
Dinner:							
Snack:							
Other Meal							
Other Meal							
Add it up:							

Circle One Daily

☺

☹

☹

Hunger Level

+ －

Exercise: (Include Videos, Walking, Exercise equipment, Any type of exercise that you did)
After exercising I felt _____
Type_____ How Long: _____
Type_____ How Long: _____
Type_____ How Long: _____
Type_____ How Long: _____

Strength Training: After working out I felt:_____

_____	X_____	Reps at _____	lbs
_____	X_____	Reps at _____	lbs
_____	X_____	Reps at _____	lbs
_____	X_____	Reps at _____	lbs
_____	X_____	Reps at _____	lbs
_____	X_____	Reps at _____	lbs
_____	X_____	Reps at _____	lbs
_____	X_____	Reps at _____	lbs

All we are given is possibilities to make of ourselves one thing or another ~
Unknown Author

Today was:

Those who say it can't be done are being passed by those doing it ~ *Unknown Author*

Daily Journal   Today's Date: _____   Weight: _____
My Mood: _____

Extra checklist boxes are to accommodate for various weight loss programs. You can check the boxes, list individual foods under Today Was page, keep a numerical log below or do all three.

Checklist: Bread/Starch: ☐☐☐☐☐☐☐☐☐, Protein: ☐☐☐☐☐☐☐☐
Veggies: ☐☐☐☐☐☐☐☐☐, Fruit: ☐☐☐☐☐☐☐☐, Fat: ☐☐☐☐☐,
Dairy: ☐☐☐☐☐☐☐☐, Water (8oz): ☐☐☐☐☐☐☐☐☐☐, Vitamin ☐

What I Ate: Protein | Fat | Carbs| Fiber |Calories| Points | Other

Breakfast: ____|____|____|____|____|____|____   Circle One
                                                    Daily
Lunch: ____|____|____|____|____|____|____
                                                    ☺
Dinner: ____|____|____|____|____|____|____
                                                    ☹
Snack: ____|____|____|____|____|____|____
                                                    ☹
Other Meal ____|____|____|____|____|____|____
                                                    Hunger Level
Other Meal ____|____|____|____|____|____|____
                                                    +   -
Add it up: ____|____|____|____|____|____|____

Exercise: (Include Videos, Walking, Exercise equipment, Any type of exercise that you did)
After exercising I felt _____
Type_____ How Long: _____
Type_____ How Long: _____
Type_____ How Long: _____
Type_____ How Long: _____

Strength Training: After working out I felt:_____

_____	X_____	Reps at _____	lbs
_____	X_____	Reps at _____	lbs
_____	X_____	Reps at _____	lbs
_____	X_____	Reps at _____	lbs
_____	X_____	Reps at _____	lbs
_____	X_____	Reps at _____	lbs
_____	X_____	Reps at _____	lbs
_____	X_____	Reps at _____	lbs

There are no shortcuts to any place worth going ~ Unknown Author

Today was:

Keep your face always toward the sunshine, and the shadows will fall behind you ~
Unknown Author

Daily Journal   Today's Date: _____   Weight: _____
My Mood: _____

Extra checklist boxes are to accommodate for various weight loss programs. You can check the boxes, list individual foods under Today Was page, keep a numerical log below or do all three.

Checklist: Bread/Starch: ☐☐☐☐☐☐☐☐, Protein: ☐☐☐☐☐☐☐☐
Veggies: ☐☐☐☐☐☐☐☐, Fruit: ☐☐☐☐☐☐☐☐, Fat: ☐☐☐☐☐,
Dairy: ☐☐☐☐☐☐☐, Water (8oz): ☐☐☐☐☐☐☐☐☐☐, Vitamin ☐

What I Ate: <u>Protein | Fat | Carbs| Fiber |Calories| Points | Other</u>

Breakfast: ____|____|____|____|____|____|____   Circle One
                                                          Daily
Lunch: ____|____|____|____|____|____|____
                                                            ☺
Dinner: ____|____|____|____|____|____|____
                                                            ☹
Snack: ____|____|____|____|____|____|____
                                                            ☹
Other Meal ____|____|____|____|____|____|____
                                                        Hunger Level
Other Meal ____|____|____|____|____|____|____
                                                           +   -
Add it up: ____|____|____|____|____|____|____

Exercise: (Include Videos, Walking, Exercise equipment, Any type of exercise that you did)
After exercising I felt _____
Type_____ How Long: _____
Type_____ How Long: _____
Type_____ How Long: _____
Type_____ How Long: _____

Strength Training: After working out I felt:_____

_____X_____	Reps at _____	lbs
_____X_____	Reps at _____	lbs
_____X_____	Reps at _____	lbs
_____X_____	Reps at _____	lbs
_____X_____	Reps at _____	lbs
_____X_____	Reps at _____	lbs
_____X_____	Reps at _____	lbs
_____X_____	Reps at _____	lbs

Life is beautiful when you burn every second doing something that matters ~
Unknown Author

Today was: _____

A smile is the light in the window of the soul indicating that the heart is home ~
Unknown Author

Daily Journal   Today's Date: _____   Weight: _____
My Mood: _____

Extra checklist boxes are to accommodate for various weight loss programs. You can check the boxes, list individual foods under Today Was page, keep a numerical log below or do all three.

Checklist: Bread/Starch: ☐☐☐☐☐☐☐☐, Protein: ☐☐☐☐☐☐☐☐
Veggies: ☐☐☐☐☐☐☐☐, Fruit: ☐☐☐☐☐☐☐☐, Fat: ☐☐☐☐☐,
Dairy: ☐☐☐☐☐☐☐, Water (8oz): ☐☐☐☐☐☐☐☐☐☐, Vitamin ☐

What I Ate: Protein | Fat | Carbs | Fiber | Calories | Points | Other

Breakfast: ____|____|____|____|____|____|____

Lunch: ____|____|____|____|____|____|____

Dinner: ____|____|____|____|____|____|____

Snack: ____|____|____|____|____|____|____

Other Meal ____|____|____|____|____|____|____

Other Meal ____|____|____|____|____|____|____

Add it up: ____|____|____|____|____|____|____

Circle One Daily

☺

😐

☹

Hunger Level

+   -

Exercise: (Include Videos, Walking, Exercise equipment, Any type of exercise that you did)
After exercising I felt _____
Type_____ How Long: _____
Type_____ How Long: _____
Type_____ How Long: _____
Type_____ How Long: _____

Strength Training: After working out I felt:_____

_____X_____	Reps at _____	lbs
_____X_____	Reps at _____	lbs
_____X_____	Reps at _____	lbs
_____X_____	Reps at _____	lbs
_____X_____	Reps at _____	lbs
_____X_____	Reps at _____	lbs
_____X_____	Reps at _____	lbs
_____X_____	Reps at _____	lbs

Life is a cup to be filled, not drained ~ Unknown Author

Today was: _____

The future belongs to those who see possibilities before they become obvious ~ Unknown Author

Daily Journal   Today's Date: _____   Weight: _____
My Mood: _____

Extra checklist boxes are to accommodate for various weight loss programs. You can check the boxes, list individual foods under Today Was page, keep a numerical log below or do all three.

Checklist: Bread/Starch: ☐ ☐ ☐ ☐ ☐ ☐ ☐ ☐, Protein: ☐ ☐ ☐ ☐ ☐ ☐ ☐ ☐
Veggies: ☐ ☐ ☐ ☐ ☐ ☐ ☐ ☐, Fruit: ☐ ☐ ☐ ☐ ☐ ☐ ☐, Fat: ☐ ☐ ☐ ☐ ☐,
Dairy: ☐ ☐ ☐ ☐ ☐ ☐ ☐, Water (8oz): ☐ ☐ ☐ ☐ ☐ ☐ ☐ ☐ ☐, Vitamin ☐

What I Ate: <u>Protein | Fat | Carbs| Fiber |Calories| Points | Other</u>

Breakfast: ____|____|____|____|____|____|____   Circle One Daily

Lunch: ____|____|____|____|____|____|____   ☺

Dinner: ____|____|____|____|____|____|____   😐

Snack: ____|____|____|____|____|____|____   ☹

Other Meal ____|____|____|____|____|____|____   Hunger Level

Other Meal ____|____|____|____|____|____|____   +   −

Add it up: ____|____|____|____|____|____|____

Exercise: (Include Videos, Walking, Exercise equipment, Any type of exercise that you did)
After exercising I felt _____
Type_____ How Long: _____
Type_____ How Long: _____
Type_____ How Long: _____
Type_____ How Long: _____

Strength Training: After working out I felt: _____

_____	X_____	Reps at _____	lbs
_____	X_____	Reps at _____	lbs
_____	X_____	Reps at _____	lbs
_____	X_____	Reps at _____	lbs
_____	X_____	Reps at _____	lbs
_____	X_____	Reps at _____	lbs
_____	X_____	Reps at _____	lbs
_____	X_____	Reps at _____	lbs

If your life is free of failures, you're not taking enough risks ~ Unknown Author

Today was:

Set your mind on a definite goal and observe how quickly the world stands aside to let you pass ~ Unknown Author

Daily Journal   Today's Date: _____   Weight: _____
My Mood: _____

Extra checklist boxes are to accommodate for various weight loss programs. You can check the boxes, list individual foods under Today Was page, keep a numerical log below or do all three.

Checklist: Bread/Starch: ☐☐☐☐☐☐☐☐, Protein: ☐☐☐☐☐☐☐☐
Veggies: ☐☐☐☐☐☐☐☐, Fruit: ☐☐☐☐☐☐☐☐, Fat: ☐☐☐☐☐☐,
Dairy: ☐☐☐☐☐☐☐☐, Water (8oz): ☐☐☐☐☐☐☐☐☐☐, Vitamin ☐

What I Ate: Protein | Fat | Carbs | Fiber | Calories | Points | Other

Breakfast: _____|_____|_____|_____|_____|_____|_____   Circle One Daily

Lunch: _____|_____|_____|_____|_____|_____|_____   ☺

Dinner: _____|_____|_____|_____|_____|_____|_____   😐

Snack: _____|_____|_____|_____|_____|_____|_____   ☹

Other Meal _____|_____|_____|_____|_____|_____|_____

Other Meal _____|_____|_____|_____|_____|_____|_____   Hunger Level

Add it up: _____|_____|_____|_____|_____|_____|_____   +   -

Exercise: (Include Videos, Walking, Exercise equipment, Any type of exercise that you did)
After exercising I felt _____
Type_____ How Long: _____
Type_____ How Long: _____
Type_____ How Long: _____
Type_____ How Long: _____

Strength Training: After working out I felt:_____

_____	X_____	Reps at _____	lbs
_____	X_____	Reps at _____	lbs
_____	X_____	Reps at _____	lbs
_____	X_____	Reps at _____	lbs
_____	X_____	Reps at _____	lbs
_____	X_____	Reps at _____	lbs
_____	X_____	Reps at _____	lbs
_____	X_____	Reps at _____	lbs

The only person you need to prove anything to is yourself ~ Unknown Author

Today was:

Follow your heart and you'll never get lost ~ Unknown Author

Daily Journal   Today's Date: _____   Weight: _____
My Mood: _____

Extra checklist boxes are to accommodate for various weight loss programs. You can check the boxes, list individual foods under Today Was page, keep a numerical log below or do all three.

Checklist: Bread/Starch: ☐☐☐☐☐☐☐☐, Protein: ☐☐☐☐☐☐☐☐
Veggies: ☐☐☐☐☐☐☐☐, Fruit: ☐☐☐☐☐☐☐☐, Fat: ☐☐☐☐☐,
Dairy: ☐☐☐☐☐☐☐☐, Water (8oz): ☐☐☐☐☐☐☐☐☐☐, Vitamin ☐

What I Ate: Protein | Fat | Carbs | Fiber | Calories | Points | Other

Breakfast: ____|____|____|____|____|____|____

Lunch: ____|____|____|____|____|____|____

Dinner: ____|____|____|____|____|____|____

Snack: ____|____|____|____|____|____|____

Other Meal ____|____|____|____|____|____|____

Other Meal ____|____|____|____|____|____|____

Add it up: ____|____|____|____|____|____|____

Circle One Daily

☺

☹

☹

Hunger Level

\+   -

Exercise: (Include Videos, Walking, Exercise equipment, Any type of exercise that you did)
After exercising I felt _____
Type_____ How Long: _____
Type_____ How Long: _____
Type_____ How Long: _____
Type_____ How Long: _____

Strength Training: After working out I felt:_____

_____	X_____	Reps at _____	lbs
_____	X_____	Reps at _____	lbs
_____	X_____	Reps at _____	lbs
_____	X_____	Reps at _____	lbs
_____	X_____	Reps at _____	lbs
_____	X_____	Reps at _____	lbs
_____	X_____	Reps at _____	lbs
_____	X_____	Reps at _____	lbs

If you expect nothing but the best you might get it ~ Unknown Author

Today was: _____

What comes around goes around~ Unknown Author

Daily Journal   Today's Date: _____   Weight: _____
My Mood: _____

Extra checklist boxes are to accommodate for various weight loss programs. You can check the boxes, list individual foods under Today Was page, keep a numerical log below or do all three.

Checklist: Bread/Starch: ☐ ☐ ☐ ☐ ☐ ☐ ☐ ☐, Protein: ☐ ☐ ☐ ☐ ☐ ☐ ☐ ☐
Veggies: ☐ ☐ ☐ ☐ ☐ ☐ ☐ ☐, Fruit: ☐ ☐ ☐ ☐ ☐ ☐ ☐ ☐, Fat: ☐ ☐ ☐ ☐ ☐ ☐,
Dairy: ☐ ☐ ☐ ☐ ☐ ☐ ☐, Water (8oz): ☐ ☐ ☐ ☐ ☐ ☐ ☐ ☐ ☐, Vitamin ☐

What I Ate: Protein | Fat | Carbs | Fiber | Calories | Points | Other

Breakfast: ___|___|___|___|___|___|___

Lunch: ___|___|___|___|___|___|___

Dinner: ___|___|___|___|___|___|___

Snack: ___|___|___|___|___|___|___

Other Meal ___|___|___|___|___|___|___

Other Meal ___|___|___|___|___|___|___

Add it up: ___|___|___|___|___|___|___

Circle One Daily

☺

☹

☹

Hunger Level

+ -

Exercise: (Include Videos, Walking, Exercise equipment, Any type of exercise that you did)
After exercising I felt _____
Type_____ How Long: _____
Type_____ How Long: _____
Type_____ How Long: _____
Type_____ How Long: _____

Strength Training: After working out I felt:_____

_____ X _____	Reps at	_____ lbs
_____ X _____	Reps at	_____ lbs
_____ X _____	Reps at	_____ lbs
_____ X _____	Reps at	_____ lbs
_____ X _____	Reps at	_____ lbs
_____ X _____	Reps at	_____ lbs
_____ X _____	Reps at	_____ lbs
_____ X _____	Reps at	_____ lbs

Think big, believe big, act big, and the results will be big ~ Unknown Author

Today was:

The greatest pleasure in life is doing what people say you cannot ~ Unknown Author

Daily Journal   Today's Date: _____   Weight: _____
My Mood: _____

Extra checklist boxes are to accommodate for various weight loss programs. You can check the boxes, list individual foods under Today Was page, keep a numerical log below or do all three.

Checklist: Bread/Starch: ☐☐☐☐☐☐☐☐, Protein: ☐☐☐☐☐☐☐☐
Veggies: ☐☐☐☐☐☐☐☐, Fruit: ☐☐☐☐☐☐☐☐, Fat: ☐☐☐☐☐,
Dairy: ☐☐☐☐☐☐☐, Water (8oz): ☐☐☐☐☐☐☐☐☐☐, Vitamin ☐

What I Ate: Protein | Fat | Carbs| Fiber |Calories| Points | Other

Breakfast: ____|____|____|____|____|____|____

Lunch: ____|____|____|____|____|____|____

Dinner: ____|____|____|____|____|____|____

Snack: ____|____|____|____|____|____|____

Other Meal ____|____|____|____|____|____|____

Other Meal ____|____|____|____|____|____|____

Add it up: ____|____|____|____|____|____|____

Circle One
Daily

☺

☹

☹

Hunger Level

+   -

Exercise: (Include Videos, Walking, Exercise equipment, Any type of exercise that you did)
After exercising I felt _____
Type_____ How Long: _____
Type_____ How Long: _____
Type_____ How Long: _____
Type_____ How Long: _____

Strength Training: After working out I felt:_____

_____ X _____	Reps at _____	lbs
_____ X _____	Reps at _____	lbs
_____ X _____	Reps at _____	lbs
_____ X _____	Reps at _____	lbs
_____ X _____	Reps at _____	lbs
_____ X _____	Reps at _____	lbs
_____ X _____	Reps at _____	lbs
_____ X _____	Reps at _____	lbs

Whoever is happy will make others happy too ~ Unknown Author

Today was: _____

The difference between a pipe dream and a great idea is persistence ~ *Unknown Author*

Daily Journal   Today's Date: _____   Weight: _____
My Mood: _____

Extra checklist boxes are to accommodate for various weight loss programs. You can check the boxes, list individual foods under Today Was page, keep a numerical log below or do all three.

Checklist: Bread/Starch: ☐☐☐☐☐☐☐☐, Protein: ☐☐☐☐☐☐☐☐
Veggies: ☐☐☐☐☐☐☐☐, Fruit: ☐☐☐☐☐☐☐☐, Fat: ☐☐☐☐☐,
Dairy: ☐☐☐☐☐☐☐, Water (8oz): ☐☐☐☐☐☐☐☐☐☐, Vitamin ☐

What I Ate: Protein | Fat | Carbs | Fiber | Calories | Points | Other

	Protein	Fat	Carbs	Fiber	Calories	Points	Other
Breakfast:							
Lunch:							
Dinner:							
Snack:							
Other Meal							
Other Meal							
Add it up:							

Circle One Daily

☺

☹

☹

Hunger Level

+   -

Exercise: (Include Videos, Walking, Exercise equipment, Any type of exercise that you did)
After exercising I felt _____
Type_____ How Long: _____
Type_____ How Long: _____
Type_____ How Long: _____
Type_____ How Long: _____

Strength Training: After working out I felt:_____

_____	X_____	Reps at _____	lbs
_____	X_____	Reps at _____	lbs
_____	X_____	Reps at _____	lbs
_____	X_____	Reps at _____	lbs
_____	X_____	Reps at _____	lbs
_____	X_____	Reps at _____	lbs
_____	X_____	Reps at _____	lbs
_____	X_____	Reps at _____	lbs

Look at life through the eyes of a child; full of wonder, love and light, then you too shall feel the joy of a day that's full and bright ~ Melissa Alvarez

Today was:

What you achieve through the journey of life is not as important as who you become ~
Unknown Author

Daily Journal Today's Date: _____   Weight: _____
My Mood: _____

Extra checklist boxes are to accommodate for various weight loss programs. You can check the boxes, list individual foods under Today Was page, keep a numerical log below or do all three.

Checklist: Bread/Starch: ☐☐☐☐☐☐☐☐, Protein: ☐☐☐☐☐☐☐☐
Veggies: ☐☐☐☐☐☐☐☐, Fruit: ☐☐☐☐☐☐☐☐, Fat: ☐☐☐☐☐,
Dairy: ☐☐☐☐☐☐☐, Water (8oz): ☐☐☐☐☐☐☐☐☐☐, Vitamin ☐

What I Ate: Protein | Fat | Carbs | Fiber | Calories | Points | Other

Breakfast: _____|_____|_____|_____|_____|_____|_____   Circle One Daily

Lunch: _____|_____|_____|_____|_____|_____|_____   ☺

Dinner: _____|_____|_____|_____|_____|_____|_____   😐

Snack: _____|_____|_____|_____|_____|_____|_____   ☹

Other Meal _____|_____|_____|_____|_____|_____|_____
                                                            Hunger Level
Other Meal _____|_____|_____|_____|_____|_____|_____
                                                            +   −
Add it up: _____|_____|_____|_____|_____|_____|_____

Exercise: (Include Videos, Walking, Exercise equipment, Any type of exercise that you did)
After exercising I felt _____
Type_____ How Long: _____
Type_____ How Long: _____
Type_____ How Long: _____
Type_____ How Long: _____

Strength Training: After working out I felt:_____

_____X_____	Reps at _____	lbs
_____X_____	Reps at _____	lbs
_____X_____	Reps at _____	lbs
_____X_____	Reps at _____	lbs
_____X_____	Reps at _____	lbs
_____X_____	Reps at _____	lbs
_____X_____	Reps at _____	lbs
_____X_____	Reps at _____	lbs

Some dream of doing great things, while others stay awake and get on with it ~
Unknown Author

Today was: _____

Time invested in improving ourselves cuts down on time wasted in disapproving of others ~ Unknown Author

Daily Journal

Today's Date: _____ Weight: _____

My Mood: _____

Extra checklist boxes are to accommodate for various weight loss programs. You can check the boxes, list individual foods under Today Was page, keep a numerical log below or do all three.

Checklist: Bread/Starch: ☐☐☐☐☐☐☐☐, Protein: ☐☐☐☐☐☐☐☐
Veggies: ☐☐☐☐☐☐☐☐, Fruit: ☐☐☐☐☐☐☐☐, Fat: ☐☐☐☐☐☐,
Dairy: ☐☐☐☐☐☐☐☐, Water (8oz): ☐☐☐☐☐☐☐☐☐☐, Vitamin ☐

What I Ate: Protein | Fat | Carbs | Fiber | Calories | Points | Other

Breakfast: _____|_____|_____|_____|_____|_____|_____

Lunch: _____|_____|_____|_____|_____|_____|_____

Dinner: _____|_____|_____|_____|_____|_____|_____

Snack: _____|_____|_____|_____|_____|_____|_____

Other Meal _____|_____|_____|_____|_____|_____|_____

Other Meal _____|_____|_____|_____|_____|_____|_____

Add it up: _____|_____|_____|_____|_____|_____|_____

Circle One Daily

☺

☹

☹

Hunger Level

+   -

Exercise: (Include Videos, Walking, Exercise equipment, Any type of exercise that you did)
After exercising I felt _____
Type_____ How Long: _____
Type_____ How Long: _____
Type_____ How Long: _____
Type_____ How Long: _____

Strength Training: After working out I felt:_____

_____	X_____	Reps at _____	lbs
_____	X_____	Reps at _____	lbs
_____	X_____	Reps at _____	lbs
_____	X_____	Reps at _____	lbs
_____	X_____	Reps at _____	lbs
_____	X_____	Reps at _____	lbs
_____	X_____	Reps at _____	lbs
_____	X_____	Reps at _____	lbs

The positive thinker sees the invisible, feels the intangible, and achieves the impossible
~ *Unknown Author*

Today was:

If you find a path with no obstacles--it is probably a path that doesn't lead anywhere
~ *Unknown Author*

Daily Journal   Today's Date: _____   Weight: _____
My Mood: _____

Extra checklist boxes are to accommodate for various weight loss programs. You can check the boxes, list individual foods under Today Was page, keep a numerical log below or do all three.

Checklist: Bread/Starch: ☐☐☐☐☐☐☐☐, Protein: ☐☐☐☐☐☐☐☐
Veggies: ☐☐☐☐☐☐☐☐, Fruit: ☐☐☐☐☐☐☐☐, Fat: ☐☐☐☐☐☐,
Dairy: ☐☐☐☐☐☐☐, Water (8oz): ☐☐☐☐☐☐☐☐☐☐, Vitamin ☐

What I Ate: Protein | Fat | Carbs| Fiber |Calories| Points | Other

Breakfast: ____|____|____|____|____|____|____   Circle One Daily

Lunch: ____|____|____|____|____|____|____   ☺

Dinner: ____|____|____|____|____|____|____   😐

Snack: ____|____|____|____|____|____|____   ☹

Other Meal ____|____|____|____|____|____|____   Hunger Level

Other Meal ____|____|____|____|____|____|____   +   −

Add it up: ____|____|____|____|____|____|____

Exercise: (Include Videos, Walking, Exercise equipment, Any type of exercise that you did)
After exercising I felt _____
Type_____ How Long: _____
Type_____ How Long: _____
Type_____ How Long: _____
Type_____ How Long: _____

Strength Training: After working out I felt:_____

_____	X_____	Reps at _____	lbs
_____	X_____	Reps at _____	lbs
_____	X_____	Reps at _____	lbs
_____	X_____	Reps at _____	lbs
_____	X_____	Reps at _____	lbs
_____	X_____	Reps at _____	lbs
_____	X_____	Reps at _____	lbs
_____	X_____	Reps at _____	lbs

Success is getting what you want, Happiness is liking what you get ~ Unknown Author

Today was: _____

Don't let fear hold you back ~ Melissa Alvarez

Daily Journal   Today's Date: _____   Weight: _____
My Mood: _____

Extra checklist boxes are to accommodate for various weight loss programs. You can check the boxes, list individual foods under Today Was page, keep a numerical log below or do all three.

Checklist: Bread/Starch: ☐☐☐☐☐☐☐☐, Protein: ☐☐☐☐☐☐☐☐
Veggies: ☐☐☐☐☐☐☐☐, Fruit: ☐☐☐☐☐☐☐☐, Fat: ☐☐☐☐☐☐,
Dairy: ☐☐☐☐☐☐☐☐, Water (8oz): ☐☐☐☐☐☐☐☐☐☐, Vitamin ☐

What I Ate: Protein | Fat | Carbs| Fiber |Calories| Points | Other

Breakfast: ____|____|____|____|____|____|____   Circle One Daily

Lunch: ____|____|____|____|____|____|____   ☺

Dinner: ____|____|____|____|____|____|____   😐

Snack: ____|____|____|____|____|____|____   ☹

Other Meal ____|____|____|____|____|____|____

Other Meal ____|____|____|____|____|____|____   Hunger Level

Add it up: ____|____|____|____|____|____|____   +   -

Exercise: (Include Videos, Walking, Exercise equipment, Any type of exercise that you did)
After exercising I felt _____
Type_____ How Long: _____
Type_____ How Long: _____
Type_____ How Long: _____
Type_____ How Long: _____

Strength Training: After working out I felt:_____

_____	X_____	Reps at _____	lbs
_____	X_____	Reps at _____	lbs
_____	X_____	Reps at _____	lbs
_____	X_____	Reps at _____	lbs
_____	X_____	Reps at _____	lbs
_____	X_____	Reps at _____	lbs
_____	X_____	Reps at _____	lbs
_____	X_____	Reps at _____	lbs

If you want to get a pail of milk, don't sit yourself on a stool in the middle of a field hoping that a cow will come over to you ~ Unknown Author

Today was:

The road to success is not doing one thing 100 percent better, but doing 100 things one percent better~ Unknown Author

Daily Journal Today's Date: _____ Weight: _____
My Mood: _____

Extra checklist boxes are to accommodate for various weight loss programs. You can check the boxes, list individual foods under Today Was page, keep a numerical log below or do all three.

Checklist: Bread/Starch: ☐☐☐☐☐☐☐☐, Protein: ☐☐☐☐☐☐☐☐
Veggies: ☐☐☐☐☐☐☐☐, Fruit: ☐☐☐☐☐☐☐☐, Fat: ☐☐☐☐☐☐,
Dairy: ☐☐☐☐☐☐☐☐, Water (8oz): ☐☐☐☐☐☐☐☐☐☐, Vitamin ☐

What I Ate: Protein | Fat | Carbs | Fiber | Calories | Points | Other

Breakfast: ____|____|____|____|____|____|____   Circle One Daily

Lunch: ____|____|____|____|____|____|____   ☺

Dinner: ____|____|____|____|____|____|____   😐

Snack: ____|____|____|____|____|____|____   ☹

Other Meal ____|____|____|____|____|____|____

Other Meal ____|____|____|____|____|____|____   Hunger Level

Add it up: ____|____|____|____|____|____|____   +   −

Exercise: (Include Videos, Walking, Exercise equipment, Any type of exercise that you did)
After exercising I felt _____
Type_____ How Long: _____
Type_____ How Long: _____
Type_____ How Long: _____
Type_____ How Long: _____

Strength Training: After working out I felt: _____

_____	X_____	Reps at _____	lbs
_____	X_____	Reps at _____	lbs
_____	X_____	Reps at _____	lbs
_____	X_____	Reps at _____	lbs
_____	X_____	Reps at _____	lbs
_____	X_____	Reps at _____	lbs
_____	X_____	Reps at _____	lbs
_____	X_____	Reps at _____	lbs

Reach high, for stars lie hidden in your soul. Dream deep, for every dream precedes the goal ~ Unknown Author

Today was:

Obstacles are put in our way to see if we really want something or we just thought we did ~ Unknown Author

Daily Journal   Today's Date: _____   Weight: _____
My Mood: _____

Extra checklist boxes are to accommodate for various weight loss programs. You can check the boxes, list individual foods under Today Was page, keep a numerical log below or do all three.

Checklist: Bread/Starch: ☐☐☐☐☐☐☐☐, Protein: ☐☐☐☐☐☐☐☐
Veggies: ☐☐☐☐☐☐☐☐, Fruit: ☐☐☐☐☐☐☐☐, Fat: ☐☐☐☐☐☐,
Dairy: ☐☐☐☐☐☐☐☐, Water (8oz): ☐☐☐☐☐☐☐☐☐☐, Vitamin ☐

What I Ate: Protein | Fat | Carbs| Fiber |Calories| Points | Other

Breakfast: ____|____|____|____|____|____|____   Circle One Daily

Lunch: ____|____|____|____|____|____|____

☺

Dinner: ____|____|____|____|____|____|____

😐

Snack: ____|____|____|____|____|____|____

☹

Other Meal ____|____|____|____|____|____|____

Other Meal ____|____|____|____|____|____|____   Hunger Level

Add it up: ____|____|____|____|____|____|____   +   -

Exercise: (Include Videos, Walking, Exercise equipment, Any type of exercise that you did)
After exercising I felt _____
Type_____ How Long: _____
Type_____ How Long: _____
Type_____ How Long: _____
Type_____ How Long: _____

Strength Training: After working out I felt:_____

_____	X_____	Reps at _____	lbs
_____	X_____	Reps at _____	lbs
_____	X_____	Reps at _____	lbs
_____	X_____	Reps at _____	lbs
_____	X_____	Reps at _____	lbs
_____	X_____	Reps at _____	lbs
_____	X_____	Reps at _____	lbs
_____	X_____	Reps at _____	lbs

To be a star, you must shine your own light, follow your own path, and don't worry about the darkness, for that is when the stars shine brightest ~ Unknown Author

Today was: _____

When BETTER is possible, then GOOD is not enough ~ Unknown Author

Daily Journal   Today's Date: _____   Weight: _____
My Mood: _____

Extra checklist boxes are to accommodate for various weight loss programs. You can check the boxes, list individual foods under Today Was page, keep a numerical log below or do all three.

Checklist: Bread/Starch: ☐☐☐☐☐☐☐☐, Protein: ☐☐☐☐☐☐☐☐
Veggies: ☐☐☐☐☐☐☐☐, Fruit: ☐☐☐☐☐☐☐☐, Fat: ☐☐☐☐☐,
Dairy: ☐☐☐☐☐☐☐, Water (8oz): ☐☐☐☐☐☐☐☐☐☐, Vitamin ☐

What I Ate: Protein | Fat | Carbs| Fiber |Calories| Points | Other

Breakfast: ____|____|____|____|____|____|____   Circle One Daily

Lunch: ____|____|____|____|____|____|____   ☺

Dinner: ____|____|____|____|____|____|____

Snack: ____|____|____|____|____|____|____   😐

Other Meal ____|____|____|____|____|____|____   ☹

Other Meal ____|____|____|____|____|____|____   Hunger Level

Add it up: ____|____|____|____|____|____|____   +   −

Exercise: (Include Videos, Walking, Exercise equipment, Any type of exercise that you did)
After exercising I felt _____
Type_____ How Long: _____
Type_____ How Long: _____
Type_____ How Long: _____
Type_____ How Long: _____

Strength Training: After working out I felt:_____

_____	X_____	Reps at _____	lbs
_____	X_____	Reps at _____	lbs
_____	X_____	Reps at _____	lbs
_____	X_____	Reps at _____	lbs
_____	X_____	Reps at _____	lbs
_____	X_____	Reps at _____	lbs
_____	X_____	Reps at _____	lbs
_____	X_____	Reps at _____	lbs

Purpose serves as a principal around which to organize our lives ~ Unknown Author

Today was:

When you delight in the game the effort seems unimportant ~ Unknown Author

Daily Journal   Today's Date: _____   Weight: _____
My Mood: _____

Extra checklist boxes are to accommodate for various weight loss programs. You can check the boxes, list individual foods under Today Was page, keep a numerical log below or do all three.

Checklist: Bread/Starch: ☐☐☐☐☐☐☐☐, Protein: ☐☐☐☐☐☐☐☐
Veggies: ☐☐☐☐☐☐☐☐, Fruit: ☐☐☐☐☐☐☐☐, Fat: ☐☐☐☐☐,
Dairy: ☐☐☐☐☐☐☐, Water (8oz): ☐☐☐☐☐☐☐☐☐☐, Vitamin ☐

What I Ate: Protein | Fat | Carbs | Fiber | Calories | Points | Other

Breakfast: _____|_____|_____|_____|_____|_____|_____

Lunch: _____|_____|_____|_____|_____|_____|_____

Dinner: _____|_____|_____|_____|_____|_____|_____

Snack: _____|_____|_____|_____|_____|_____|_____

Other Meal _____|_____|_____|_____|_____|_____|_____

Other Meal _____|_____|_____|_____|_____|_____|_____

Add it up: _____|_____|_____|_____|_____|_____|_____

Circle One Daily

☺

☐ (neutral face)

☹

Hunger Level

+   -

Exercise: (Include Videos, Walking, Exercise equipment, Any type of exercise that you did)
After exercising I felt _____
Type_____ How Long: _____
Type_____ How Long: _____
Type_____ How Long: _____
Type_____ How Long: _____

Strength Training: After working out I felt:_____

_____X_____	Reps at _____	lbs
_____X_____	Reps at _____	lbs
_____X_____	Reps at _____	lbs
_____X_____	Reps at _____	lbs
_____X_____	Reps at _____	lbs
_____X_____	Reps at _____	lbs
_____X_____	Reps at _____	lbs
_____X_____	Reps at _____	lbs

A smile costs you nothing. It's a little thing, but will always produce big results ~
Unknown Author

Today was:

Footprints on the sands of time are never made by sitting down ~ Unknown Author

Daily Journal   Today's Date: _____   Weight: _____
My Mood: _____

Extra checklist boxes are to accommodate for various weight loss programs. You can check the boxes, list individual foods under Today Was page, keep a numerical log below or do all three.

Checklist: Bread/Starch: ☐☐☐☐☐☐☐☐, Protein: ☐☐☐☐☐☐☐☐
Veggies: ☐☐☐☐☐☐☐☐, Fruit: ☐☐☐☐☐☐☐☐, Fat: ☐☐☐☐☐☐,
Dairy: ☐☐☐☐☐☐☐, Water (8oz): ☐☐☐☐☐☐☐☐☐☐, Vitamin ☐

What I Ate: <u>Protein | Fat | Carbs| Fiber |Calories| Points | Other</u>

Breakfast: ____|____|____|____|____|____|____   Circle One
                                                        Daily
Lunch: ____|____|____|____|____|____|____
                                                          ☺
Dinner: ____|____|____|____|____|____|____
                                                          ☺
Snack: ____|____|____|____|____|____|____
                                                          ☹
Other Meal ____|____|____|____|____|____|____
                                                       Hunger Level
Other Meal ____|____|____|____|____|____|____
                                                          + -
Add it up: ____|____|____|____|____|____|____

Exercise: (Include Videos, Walking, Exercise equipment, Any type of exercise that you did)
After exercising I felt _____
Type_____ How Long: _____
Type_____ How Long: _____
Type_____ How Long: _____
Type_____ How Long: _____

Strength Training: After working out I felt:_____

_____	X_____	Reps at _____	lbs
_____	X_____	Reps at _____	lbs
_____	X_____	Reps at _____	lbs
_____	X_____	Reps at _____	lbs
_____	X_____	Reps at _____	lbs
_____	X_____	Reps at _____	lbs
_____	X_____	Reps at _____	lbs
_____	X_____	Reps at _____	lbs

You can make good choices, you can make rotten choices, but you can make choices ~
Unknown Author

Today was:

It's not the obstacle we conquer, but ourselves ~ Unknown Author

Daily Journal   Today's Date: _____   Weight: _____
My Mood: _____

Extra checklist boxes are to accommodate for various weight loss programs. You can check the boxes, list individual foods under Today Was page, keep a numerical log below or do all three.

Checklist: Bread/Starch: ☐☐☐☐☐☐☐☐, Protein: ☐☐☐☐☐☐☐☐
Veggies: ☐☐☐☐☐☐☐☐, Fruit: ☐☐☐☐☐☐☐☐, Fat: ☐☐☐☐☐,
Dairy: ☐☐☐☐☐☐☐, Water (8oz): ☐☐☐☐☐☐☐☐☐☐, Vitamin ☐

What I Ate: Protein | Fat | Carbs | Fiber | Calories | Points | Other

Breakfast: ____|____|____|____|____|____|____   Circle One Daily

Lunch: ____|____|____|____|____|____|____   ☺

Dinner: ____|____|____|____|____|____|____   😐

Snack: ____|____|____|____|____|____|____   ☹

Other Meal ____|____|____|____|____|____|____   Hunger Level

Other Meal ____|____|____|____|____|____|____   +   -

Add it up: ____|____|____|____|____|____|____

Exercise: (Include Videos, Walking, Exercise equipment, Any type of exercise that you did)
After exercising I felt _____
Type_____ How Long: _____
Type_____ How Long: _____
Type_____ How Long: _____
Type_____ How Long: _____

Strength Training: After working out I felt:_____

_____	X _____	Reps at _____	lbs
_____	X _____	Reps at _____	lbs
_____	X _____	Reps at _____	lbs
_____	X _____	Reps at _____	lbs
_____	X _____	Reps at _____	lbs
_____	X _____	Reps at _____	lbs
_____	X _____	Reps at _____	lbs
_____	X _____	Reps at _____	lbs

There will never be another now, so I will make the most of today. There will never be another me, so I will make the most of myself ~ Unknown Author

Today was: _____

Challenges can be stepping stones or stumbling blocks. It's just a matter of how you view them ~ Unknown Author

Daily Journal   Today's Date: _____   Weight: _____
My Mood: _____

Extra checklist boxes are to accommodate for various weight loss programs. You can check the boxes, list individual foods under Today Was page, keep a numerical log below or do all three.

Checklist: Bread/Starch: ☐☐☐☐☐☐☐☐☐, Protein: ☐☐☐☐☐☐☐☐
Veggies: ☐☐☐☐☐☐☐☐, Fruit: ☐☐☐☐☐☐☐☐, Fat: ☐☐☐☐☐☐,
Dairy: ☐☐☐☐☐☐☐☐, Water (8oz): ☐☐☐☐☐☐☐☐☐☐, Vitamin ☐

What I Ate: Protein | Fat | Carbs | Fiber | Calories | Points | Other

Meal	Protein	Fat	Carbs	Fiber	Calories	Points	Other
Breakfast:							
Lunch:							
Dinner:							
Snack:							
Other Meal							
Other Meal							
Add it up:							

Circle One Daily

☺

☹ (neutral)

☹ (sad)

Hunger Level

\+   −

Exercise: (Include Videos, Walking, Exercise equipment, Any type of exercise that you did)
After exercising I felt _____
Type_____ How Long: _____
Type_____ How Long: _____
Type_____ How Long: _____
Type_____ How Long: _____

Strength Training: After working out I felt: _____

_____	X_____	Reps at _____	lbs
_____	X_____	Reps at _____	lbs
_____	X_____	Reps at _____	lbs
_____	X_____	Reps at _____	lbs
_____	X_____	Reps at _____	lbs
_____	X_____	Reps at _____	lbs
_____	X_____	Reps at _____	lbs
_____	X_____	Reps at _____	lbs

Your vision will become clear only when you look into your heart, those who look outside DREAM, those who look inside AWAKEN ~ Unknown Author

Today was:

No one can choose your mountain or tell you when to climb It's yours alone to challenge at your own pace and time~ Unknown Author

Daily Journal Today's Date: _____ Weight: _____
My Mood: _____

Extra checklist boxes are to accommodate for various weight loss programs. You can check the boxes, list individual foods under Today Was page, keep a numerical log below or do all three.

Checklist: Bread/Starch: ☐☐☐☐☐☐☐☐, Protein: ☐☐☐☐☐☐☐☐
Veggies: ☐☐☐☐☐☐☐☐, Fruit: ☐☐☐☐☐☐☐☐, Fat: ☐☐☐☐☐☐,
Dairy: ☐☐☐☐☐☐☐☐, Water (8oz): ☐☐☐☐☐☐☐☐☐☐, Vitamin ☐

What I Ate: <u>Protein | Fat | Carbs| Fiber |Calories| Points | Other</u>

Breakfast: ____|____|____|____|____|____|____

Lunch: ____|____|____|____|____|____|____

Dinner: ____|____|____|____|____|____|____

Snack: ____|____|____|____|____|____|____

Other Meal ____|____|____|____|____|____|____

Other Meal ____|____|____|____|____|____|____

Add it up: ____|____|____|____|____|____|____

Circle One Daily

☺

😐

☹

Hunger Level

+   -

Exercise: (Include Videos, Walking, Exercise equipment, Any type of exercise that you did)
After exercising I felt _____
Type_____ How Long: _____
Type_____ How Long: _____
Type_____ How Long: _____
Type_____ How Long: _____

Strength Training: After working out I felt:_____

_____	X_____	Reps at _____	lbs
_____	X_____	Reps at _____	lbs
_____	X_____	Reps at _____	lbs
_____	X_____	Reps at _____	lbs
_____	X_____	Reps at _____	lbs
_____	X_____	Reps at _____	lbs
_____	X_____	Reps at _____	lbs
_____	X_____	Reps at _____	lbs

If you have discipline, you can conquer the world. If you don't have discipline, the world will conquer you ~ Unknown Author

Today was: _____

Do not follow where the path may lead, go instead where there is no path and leave a trail ~ Unknown Author

Daily Journal   Today's Date: _____   Weight: _____
My Mood: _____

Extra checklist boxes are to accommodate for various weight loss programs. You can check the boxes, list individual foods under Today Was page, keep a numerical log below or do all three.

Checklist: Bread/Starch: ☐☐☐☐☐☐☐☐, Protein: ☐☐☐☐☐☐☐☐
Veggies: ☐☐☐☐☐☐☐☐, Fruit: ☐☐☐☐☐☐☐☐, Fat: ☐☐☐☐☐☐,
Dairy: ☐☐☐☐☐☐☐☐, Water (8oz): ☐☐☐☐☐☐☐☐☐☐, Vitamin ☐

What I Ate: Protein | Fat | Carbs| Fiber |Calories| Points | Other

Breakfast: ____|____|____|____|____|____|____

Lunch: ____|____|____|____|____|____|____

Dinner: ____|____|____|____|____|____|____

Snack: ____|____|____|____|____|____|____

Other Meal ____|____|____|____|____|____|____

Other Meal ____|____|____|____|____|____|____

Add it up: ____|____|____|____|____|____|____

Circle One Daily

☺

☐

☹

Hunger Level

+   −

Exercise: (Include Videos, Walking, Exercise equipment, Any type of exercise that you did)
After exercising I felt _____
Type_____ How Long: _____
Type_____ How Long: _____
Type_____ How Long: _____
Type_____ How Long: _____

Strength Training: After working out I felt:_____

_____	X_____	Reps at _____	lbs
_____	X_____	Reps at _____	lbs
_____	X_____	Reps at _____	lbs
_____	X_____	Reps at _____	lbs
_____	X_____	Reps at _____	lbs
_____	X_____	Reps at _____	lbs
_____	X_____	Reps at _____	lbs
_____	X_____	Reps at _____	lbs

YOU DID IT!!!

CONGRATULATIONS ON YOUR SUCCESS!!!

You have looked deep inside and from your inner self, your strength and desires, have transformed yourself just like the Phoenix.

I applaud you!!!

GREAT JOB!!!

VISIT MELISSA ALVAREZ ONLINE AT
www.MelissaA.com

Email Melissa at
contact@melissaa.com